Yoga students everywhere will be grateful for Charlotte Bell's thoughtful guidance through the path of classical yoga. Her book is packed with stories that help us make sense of the sometimes-complex teachings of this ancient technique—and the practical quality of her wisdom is irresistible.

—Stephen Cope, author of *The Wisdom of Yoga: A Seeker's Guide to Extraordinary Living*

In *Mindful Yoga, Mindful Life*, Charlotte Bell weaves in her deep personal life experiences to give the reader a comprehensive guide to a spiritual practice that is captivating and down to earth. With her many years of yoga practice and vipassana meditation, she comprehensively compares Patanjali's Yoga Sutras, including the eight limbs of yoga, with Buddhist philosophy and shows how each philosophy and practice support each other. Charlotte also has an extensive musical background and brings a lyrical quality into her writing that is creative and compelling. I highly recommend this book to my students and all students of yoga who want to explore yoga in all walks of their lives.

—Elise Browning Miller, coauthor of *Yoga: Anytime, Anywhere*

Mindful Yoga, Mindful Life is an open invitation to bring yoga to your life. Drawing on many years of yoga study, Charlotte Bell presents its core teachings, artfully weaving in personal stories from her own journey. Part memoir, part instruction, the result is a warm and accessible guidebook to be sampled, savored, and shared. Receive this book as a gift, whether you are just beginning yoga or have been on the path for years.

—Yael Calhoun, coauthor of *Create a Yoga Practice for Kids: Fun, Flexibility, and Focus*

In this intensely personal book, Charlotte Bell's life stories flow seamlessly into a thoughtful discussion of the yoga philosophy that has shaped and supported her daily life for decades. While seemingly simple, the book radiates wisdom, humor, and hope. Highly recommended for all levels of students of yoga.

—Judith Hanson Lasater, Ph.D., P.T., author of
A Year of Living Your Yoga: Daily Practices to Shape Your Life

Before I knew Charlotte Bell, I knew of' Charlotte Bell. Her impeccable reputation and high standards seemed legendary to me. Then I met her and found her to be an ordinary person living an extraordinary life. I am thrilled that she decided to write about it in this book. This book is a story of the way one woman has authentically and powerfully woven the eight limbs of yoga into her very busy Western life. This book is an invitation. It invites us to explore the Yoga Sutras as a means of exploring our own busy and sometimes confusing lives. This book is a how-to manual. It gives us practical suggestions on how to reap the benefits of yoga without giving up the world we live in. Ultimately this book is a tribute, to all of us who have ever wondered where the "yoga industry" is headed, who see yoga being branded, owned, and made exclusive, and who see self-proclaimed gurus taking credit for another person's growth. Charlotte reassures us that the true spirit and power of yoga will prevail.

—D'ana Baptiste, Director of Centered City Yoga, Salt Lake City, Utah

Mindful Yoga, Mindful Life

MINDFUL YOGA

A GUIDE FOR EVERYDAY PRACTICE

MINDFUL LIFE

CHARLOTTE BELL

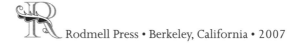
Rodmell Press • Berkeley, California • 2007

For my mother

Mindful Yoga, Mindful Life: A Guide for Everyday Practice,
copyright © 2007 by Charlotte Bell.
Cover photograph by Jose Luis Pelaez, Inc./Getty Images.
All rights reserved.

An earlier version of chapter 3 and parts of chapters 1 and 4 appeared in *Catalyst* and in *New York Spirit*.

Library of Congress
Cataloging-in-Publication Data

Bell, Charlotte, 1955-
  Mindful yoga, mindful life : a guide for everyday practice / Charlotte Bell. — 1st ed.
    p. cm.
  Includes bibliographical references and index.
  ISBN 978-1-930485-20-4 (pbk. : alk. paper)
  1. Yoga. 2. Attention. I. Title.
  B132.Y6B4225 2007
  181'.45—dc22

                          2007026732

Printed and bound in China
First Edition
ISBN-10 1-930485-20-4
ISBN-13 978-1-930485-20-4

12 11 10 09 08 07   1 2 3 4 5 6 7 8 9 10

Editor: Linda Cogozzo
Associate Editor: Holly Hammond
Indexer: Ty Koontz
Cover and Text Design: Gopa & Ted2, Inc.
Author Photographer: Roz Newmark
Lithographer: Kwong Fat Offset Printing Co., Ltd.
Text set in Joanna 11/14.5

Distributed by Publishers Group West

Contents

Acknowledgments

N O BOOK is the work of a single person. Every person I've encountered, every experience I've lived, has contributed to this text. It is with immense gratitude that I acknowledge the individuals who have helped most directly with the birth of this book, through their writing expertise, the strength of their yoga and meditation practice, or their continued support.

A community of fantastic writers have provided a solid sounding board for this project: Dawn Marano, for making my proposal shine; Dorothee Kocks, for her sage advice on the world of publishing; and Yael Calhoun, for her expertise on the process, from querying to copyediting. I am grateful for a renewed friendship with my childhood writing companion, Chandra Mattingly, whose astute eye for detail helped me refine my text when I could no longer see it for having read it so many times.

Thanks also to Greta deJong, founder of *Catalyst* magazine, who gave me my first opportunity to write for the public, and to Paul English, for the generous gift of a regular column in *New York Spirit* magazine. Finally, many thanks to Linda Cogozzo, copublisher at Rodmell Press, for so many lovely conversations and for believing in this project enough to bring it to fruition.

I've been fortunate to study yoga and meditation with teachers of incredible depth and unflagging integrity. Pujari and Abhilasha of the Last Resort have been my lifeline through virtually all the trials and triumphs of my adult life. I cannot imagine who I would be without their love, support, and guidance. Donna Farhi's teaching has expanded my practice in ways that continue to surprise me. Her writing is an inspiration, and her friendship is a jewel in my life. I am grateful to many other teachers who have shaped my understanding of yoga: Judith Hanson Lasater, Cita Mason, David Riley, Mary Dunn, and Elise Browning Miller. Thank you to Joseph Goldstein, Sharon Salzberg, Michele McDonald, Jack Kornfield, and Christina Feldman. Thanks also to Sara Chambers and the staff at Hugger-Mugger Yoga Products for two decades of inspiration, collaboration, and friendship. Finally, I am infinitely grateful to and humbled by the community of exceptional people who attend my classes each week.

Many of the stories in this book were written into my life by my birth family: my mother, Mary Jane; my father, the late Bob Bell; and my sisters, Martha and Anne. I'm ever grateful for their creativity, intelligence, and integrity. Throughout the writing process, four precocious felines—Jazzy, Pushkin, the late, great Cleocatra, and Fiona the heart kitty—have kept me balanced and have brightened my attitude with their love, loyalty, and countless humor breaks. And I am immeasurably grateful to Phillip for his love, optimism, support, and encouragement throughout the process of writing this book.

Foreword

BY DONNA FARHI

OVER TWENTY YEARS ago, I met Charlotte Bell at one of the first yoga intensives I taught in Jackson Hole, Wyoming. The deep level of introspection I sensed in her struck me. But there was something more—a recognition that she was on the cusp of some momentous change. She invited me to come and teach in her hometown, Salt Lake City, Utah, and we began a long association that continues to this day. I must admit that in those early years I was not always comfortable around Charlotte.

As she so honestly reveals in this book, she was facing huge psychological and emotional obstacles (as was I), and I found her quite a depressing and sad person to be with. Perhaps this is a strange way to begin a foreword to this wonderful book, but this information about who Charlotte was when I met her seems most important of all to me. For in the years to come, as she committed herself to one long meditation retreat after another and to her yoga practice, I was deeply privileged to witness one of the most complete metamorphoses of any person, friend or student, I had seen. Soon I looked forward to my visits with Charlotte, as she revealed a character of complete integrity. Her commitment to leading a compassionate yet at the same time inclusively human life is expressed in her sense of fun and sharply observant wit. Does yoga work? It is one thing to ask this question when everything is going our way; it is quite another thing to ask whether this centuries-old practice holds up when our life is going to hell. Charlotte decisively answers this question in Mindful Yoga, Mindful Life through sharing the trials and triumph of her own yogic journey.

Using the Yoga Sutras of Patanjali and the eight-limbed path of Ashtanga Yoga as her structural thread, Charlotte leads us into a deep exploration of what it means to lead a yogic life. She offers a fresh perspective on each sutra and limb that is at once pragmatic and relevant to the Western practitioner. As anyone who has ever attempted to study the sutras will know, Patanjali offers us a skeletal structure from which to understand the inner scaffolding of yoga philosophy. He gives us the map, but this is not the territory. One can only truly understand these sutras by a literal fleshing out of their meaning through consistent practice over the course of a lifetime, through testing each proposition, each practice, in the often less than conducive conditions of daily life. Patanjali doesn't offer us an easy or simple solution, but as Sanskrit scholar Vyaas Houston maintains, he does offer us "the certainty of freedom." What we have in this book is an insightful reflection of an understanding of yoga gleaned from direct experience. Noticeably absent in the book is the jargon of New Age cliché or generic definitions of consciousness lacking substance. Instead, you'll find a thoughtful and easily comprehended guide for navigating the territory itself.

While there is a clear and cumulative building of knowledge in this book, you can also open to any chapter and reflect on its meaning. I encourage you to read this book slowly, as if it were itself a meditation, and to return again and again to those chapters with which you resonate. Pause frequently to give yourself time to reflect on how this wisdom is relevant to you, and how you might best apply this knowledge in creating a happier and more peaceful life for yourself and for those around you.

This book comes at a time when we desperately need this kind of honest self-reflection and a deeper commitment to practices that help us come to terms with the causes of our own suffering. It comes at a time when individually and collectively we need to become clear about core values that can create conditions for a sustainable and durable future. It is a heroic journey, in which all living beings can share in the benefits of our practice.

Preface

fiRST BECAME AWARE of yoga while watching a TV commercial in the late 1960s. I don't recall what was being advertised, since I saw the commercial only once, but I still remember the image of a lithe, dark-haired woman, wearing a classic, scoop-necked, black dance leotard—the only yoga wear available in those days. I especially remember her beatific smile as she effortlessly slid her ankle behind her head, all the while speaking softly and convincingly about whatever product she was selling.

The image of the TV yogi's grace and poise stayed with me however, and in the early 1980s I decided to find a yoga class. Maybe even I could develop the kind of grace I'd admired in that long-ago commercial. By the end of the very first class, I felt a sense of inner equilibrium that brought a whole new dimension to my elementary understanding of yoga. I now understood that the lovely, fluid movements of the TV yogi came from something more than her extraordinary flexibility or finely honed technique; it was arising from inside, inseparable from the mind that produced that beatific smile. I felt as if I'd come home. I knew this practice would be with me for life.

I dove into yoga with a level of commitment I had never given to anything else. I attended as many classes and workshops as I could, and I apprenticed with my local teachers with the idea that I might someday know enough to teach. Ready or not, that day came four and a half years into my practice, when my teachers moved out of state. By then I'd developed what I thought was an impressive repertoire of techniques, and what I now know to be a fairly rudimentary understanding of the physical aspect of yoga. Two decades of dedicated practice later, I am inspired by how much there still is to learn.

The longer I practice, the more I see how vast is the territory yet to be explored. After twenty-five years of yoga practice, I feel I've just begun to comprehend the scope of yoga. When practiced with its original intent, yoga is not simply a way to keep fit. It is inseparable from the way I live my life.

Amazing feats of physical accomplishment on the yoga mat, when severed from the comprehensive system of yoga from which they spring, are little more than acrobatics. Exciting mental tricks are not the point of practice either. The place where the quality of our yoga practice speaks most clearly is in the way we live our lives. Yoga manifests in the timbre of our interactions with our friends, family, coworkers, and most of all, the people we find to be difficult.

When we give ourselves fully and consciously to our daily endeavors, we are practicing yoga. Over time, yoga enters our cells and becomes our foundation, a quality of peace that infuses everything we do. Yoga provides the ballast we need when our lives seem to be falling apart. It allows us to respond skillfully and compassionately to the countless and inevitable highs and lows of living in this world.

Some three thousand years ago, a sage named Patanjali gathered the universal wisdom of millennia into a book of verses called the Yoga Sutras. A comprehensive guide to the entire system of yoga, the sutras explore everything from ethical guidelines and worldly practices to stages of enlightenment. I have chosen one small section of the Yoga Sutras, the eight limbs of yoga, to discuss in this book. The eight limbs comprise the how-to part of the Yoga Sutras. They form a framework for applying the principles of yoga to our everyday lives.

This book was a real labor of love, probably something I've been writing half my life without ever actually getting it down on paper. My hope is that it will be useful as a springboard to your own explorations. May the timeless wisdom of yoga bring peace, joy, and wisdom to your life.

Introduction:
Stepping onto the Path

I N JUNE OF 1980, I took my first trip west of the Mississippi. A recent graduate of Indiana University, I had decided to relocate to live with a man who would become my partner for the next nine years and continues to be a friend. Moving to the great, unknown West after living my entire twenty-five years in Indiana felt like a grand adventure. I stuffed my Toyota Celica with those possessions most salient to survival and began an intrepid journey to new, unimaginable territory.

A few days before my departure, I was downtown finishing up business when an interesting person caught my eye. A red-haired man dressed entirely in orange—gym shorts, tank top, and walking shoes—strode into the town square. I remembered reading in the newspaper that a man who was walking solo across the United States to raise money for the World Hunger Project would be trekking through my town, Bloomington, Indiana, on that day. Here he was. That's cool, I thought.

I did not think about the orange-clad long-distance walker again until six years later. Four years into a committed yoga practice, I decided to attend a weeklong retreat at the Last Resort Retreat Center in Cedar Breaks, Utah. I had met the teachers, Pujari and Abhilasha Keays, a year earlier and felt immediately drawn to their work.

On the last evening of the retreat, Pujari presented a narrated slide show of a journey he had taken in 1980—a solo walk across America to raise funds for the World Hunger Project. As soon as I saw the slide of Pujari being interviewed by the media on Bloomington's town square, I not only recognized the red-haired walker I'd seen so many years before, but I knew I had stumbled upon the teacher I needed to meet.

In the subsequent decades of my practice, Pujari and his wife Abhilasha have accompanied me, one step at a time, on a surprising journey that has led me to places I could never have imagined. Along the way, I've found that the happiness that had eluded me throughout my life, perpetually pacing an elusive three steps ahead, is in reality never apart from me. All I needed to do was stop chasing after it.

The quest for happiness is universal. There is not a single being on this earth who does not seek to live a happy life. Many of us seek happiness through acquisition—of material wealth, public acknowledgment, or extraordinary experiences. Many of us seek contentment through our relationships with family, friends, and life partners. The search can take the form of devotion to an exemplary deity, as in Judeo-Christian and Islamic systems. Other seekers have sought peace through the exploration and understanding of the Self, in systems such as Buddhism. No matter what the method, the impulse is the same. All beings want to be happy.

We who have embarked on the path of yoga also do so in search of happiness. Whether we hope to find happiness in the form of a more sculpted and flexible body, or whether we long to dwell in the peace of *samadhi*, the endeavor to find contentment is the motivation.

The quest for spiritual happiness begins with some sort of inspiration. In his book *Hero with a Thousand Faces*, Joseph Campbell calls the source of spiritual inspiration the "call to destiny." This call can happen at any time in our lives. The call can be triggered by a specific event that shifts us into a new understanding, one that inspires us to look more deeply for the causes of lasting happiness. Often the call jolts us from a state of complacency. Sometimes it causes us to turn our lives in a completely unpredictable direction. For some people the call is continuous, evolving slowly over a lifetime. For others, there are many calls that define the trajectory of their paths.

One of the best-known archetypal tales of the call to destiny is the story of the Buddha, a man who achieved enlightenment nearly three thousand years ago. The Buddha's call to destiny took place early in his life. Siddhartha was born into a royal family, the prince of a small Indian kingdom. At the time of his birth, a seer predicted that he would become either a king or an *arhat*, a fully enlightened being. His father, the king, wished his son to follow in his footsteps and become the next ruler of his kingdom. He surrounded the young prince with opulence, all the earthly delights he could possibly desire, hoping to show him the pleasures of a life of power and wealth. Siddhartha was constantly entertained by a parade of musicians, dancers, and voluptuous concubines. He ate only the most exotic foods and wore only the finest silks. The king showered his son with these pleasures so that he would never desire to leave the royal life.

Still, one day Siddhartha decided he would like to venture outside his paradise. A chariot was called, and the prince set out to see the world. Before Siddhartha left, the king ordered that all signs of poverty and other unpleasantness be hidden from his view. But despite the king's best efforts, Siddhartha was confronted by the Four Heavenly Messengers who would call him to his true destiny. On his journey he saw an aged man, a man consumed with illness, and the body of a man who had died. His charioteer explained that all these conditions were natural stages in each person's life, that no one ultimately escaped old age, sickness, and death. Having never been exposed to such unpleasant realities, the young prince was profoundly affected by his discoveries. He began to question the culture of pleasure and acquisition. If we are all subject to old age, sickness, and death, what is the point of chasing after material pleasures? Where is lasting happiness to be found?

The fourth messenger the young prince saw was a monk. The charioteer told Siddhartha that this was a man who had renounced worldly life in search of a more lasting happiness. The experience of seeing these four messengers awakened in the young prince the desire to seek the kind of happiness that is not subject to the vagaries of life.

He renounced his life of royalty and spent the next six years as a monk, practicing meditation and austerities. During this time, he subjected his body to extreme deprivation, so much so that he became emaciated. Eventually he realized that neither extreme—the life of worldly desire or the life of extreme deprivation—was the way to happiness. He set out on what he called the middle way. One night, while sitting in deep meditation under the bodhi tree, he reached full enlightenment. He spent the rest of his life sharing the wisdom of his enlightenment and inspiring others to follow their own paths to awakening.

Profound life changes often inspire major reassessments. In the mid-1990s, I taught yoga for several years at the Cancer Wellness House in Salt Lake City, a community resource for cancer patients and their families. During my years of practice there, I encountered innumerable cancer survivors who said that the experience of facing their possible demise from cancer had irrevocably changed them. Most said the experience caused them to reassess their lives. Many conducted "spring cleanings," in which they freed their lives of material goods and commitments that they realized were unimportant so they could reorient themselves to what they considered to be their true callings.

One does not have to encounter death, however, to be called to awaken. My own call to destiny unfolded gradually and continues to unfold. I grew up in a largely nonreligious family. We attended a weekly service at a Presbyterian church because my father and mother, both classical vocalists, conducted and sang in the choir. We never said grace before meals and did not pray at bedtime. My mother later told me that she and my father were agnostic, a fact they had shared with our minister. He was a respectful and open-minded man—an advocate of Transcendental Meditation—and he appreciated their musical participation in his services all the same.

In church I heard lots of talk of salvation and inspiration and read scriptures that warned of a wrathful and unforgiving God. Hymns and responsive readings spoke of humankind's predicament, that we are all hopeless sinners. The way to salvation was through acceptance of Christ as savior. Even when I was quite young, I felt oddly removed from the church's philosophy. I did not feel that I was born a sinner and did not feel a need to be saved. While I observed others deriving great meaning from the teachings, I felt disconnected and sometimes even suffocated in the church. I knew that I was supposed to feel a sense of wonder, magic, and gratitude, but the Biblical stories (with the exception of the story of St. Francis, which resonated with my love of animals) seemed unrelated to my life.

I was, however, familiar with a vastness of mind that seemed beyond anything I felt in the church. I experienced this vastness when I walked in the woods behind our house. I felt it when I played piano. It was present in the stars and in the large flocks of migrating birds that blackened the sky each autumn. I entered into the vastness sitting alone on the front stoop of our house at dusk.

When I was thirteen, I was invited to join the church. This involved attending communicants' classes—weekly meetings with the minister. I attended these classes and completed whatever assignments were given. My participation was half-hearted at best. I was simply doing what I was expected to do. Everyone joined the church when they reached the end of eighth grade.

During this time I developed a pattern of insomnia. Sleepless nights were quite common for me and were mostly dominated by obsessive worry. One night, however, I began experiencing what felt like transmissions from somewhere outside myself. A flood of insight began pouring into my mind. I viewed the cycles of life from a vantage point outside my normal conscious state. I saw that we do not live just this one life and, depending on whether we were good or bad, believers or nonbelievers, we end up in Heaven or Hell. I saw that we live countless lifetimes, and with each one we gain more and more wisdom through our experiences. I saw that each time we return we refine our lives until, at some point, our spirits become so clear that we do not reincarnate. I understood that we are not born sinners. Instead, we come into this life carrying the accumulated wisdom and experience from previous lifetimes, and it is neither good nor bad. I saw that there is no fearsome God somewhere up in the sky, chalking up good deeds and bad, in order to calculate where my disembodied soul would spend eternity. I realized that the quality of my life, and my death and rebirth, were entirely up to me. I knew my happiness or unhappiness in this life and the next depended on my own choices and actions.

This insight was incredibly freeing for me. I was inspired in a way I had never been before. I knew that this understanding was my truth. Still, I told no one. I continued my classes at the church. Now the teachings felt like an interesting academic lesson. I had come home to myself on that sleepless night, and it no longer mattered that I felt misaligned with the church. I knew that the philosophy of reincarnation was incongruous with Christian thought. Since almost everyone I knew in my southern Indiana hometown was a member of one of a half dozen churches, I felt it best to keep quiet about what I now understood.

I attended Indiana University in the 1970s. While working toward a degree in Italian language—which I never deluded myself into thinking would land me a lucrative job—I paid most of my expenses by working two serving jobs. I felt fortunate to work in two of Bloomington's most venerable gathering places, Mother Bear's Pizza Barn and the Bluebird, a wild and smoky tavern that hosted an amazing array of legendary artists, luminaries such as Muddy Waters, Vassar Clements, Dizzy Gillespie, and Sun Ra. In retrospect, working as a server was probably more crucial to my evolution than the classes I attended. I was born an introvert; dealing with the public drew me out and taught me how to be comfortable with unfamiliar people. This would serve me well as I settled into my chosen profession years later.

Indiana University in the 1970s was fertile ground for experimentation with alcohol, marijuana, cocaine, and hallucinogens such as LSD and psilocybin mushrooms. I had no qualms about trying them (and I did inhale). I enjoyed the way these substances catapulted me out of my normal, seemingly stultified state of mind. I especially enjoyed the effects of hallucinogens. I loved the shift of priorities that invariably took place under their influence. Suddenly the day-to-day desires and worries that usually seemed so overwhelming became minute compared to the larger state of being I was enjoying.

During this period, one late-night conversation—a drug-induced philosophical frenzy with a friend—revealed that the insight I'd carried with me for the previous ten years was aligned with Buddhist thought. I was heartened that what I had thought was my philosophy was not simply my own invention.

After graduation, I married and moved west to Las Vegas. I settled into work as a printer in a custom photo lab and enjoyed the partnership of my marriage. In January of 1982, I decided to take a yoga class. I had long been curious about yoga but had not been in a place, physically or mentally, where I wanted to make it a priority. I began classes at June Bains Academy of Yoga. June Bains was a devotee of Sathya Sai Baba and a longtime student of the late Indra Devi. Her Indian name was Laxmi, and her classes were liberally sprinkled with Baba's and Devi's philosophies and wisdom.

Yoga practice changed my life completely. I became less interested in altering my consciousness through drugs. Yoga was showing me places in my consciousness I had never known. I felt a sense of spaciousness during and after the classes' final relaxation that was more profoundly satisfying than any experiences I had had on hallucinogens.

Within three weeks of joining the yoga class, I knew I wanted to teach. This was an odd sensation for me. I had always been extremely shy about being in front of people, so I had never considered teaching as a career. Yet the call to yoga was so strong that I felt no trepidation about teaching. The call transcended logic and previous psychological patterns. But I knew that there was a whole lot more I needed to learn before I would feel comfortable offering this precious jewel to others. The level of respect I felt for yoga was so profound that I felt a great responsibility to offer it from a place of knowledge.

When we moved to Salt Lake City four months after my introduction to yoga, I met Cita Mason and David Riley, who taught yoga in the tradition of B. K. S. Iyengar. For the next four years, I apprenticed with them, attending and assisting in their classes and meeting outside class to practice. They taught me volumes about the workings of the body and the intricacies of asana practice. They also set contrasting but equally inspiring examples of how to be a teacher.

Cita and David knew a great many yoga teachers in other locales, whom they invited to Salt Lake to teach intensive workshops. In reflecting on that four-year period, I feel fortunate to have studied with so many different teachers—inspired yogis like Judith Hanson Lasater, Mary Dunn, Roger Cole, Jean Couch, Felicity Green, Ramanand Patel, and Pujari—in relatively intimate classes of twenty to thirty students.

In 1986 Cita and David moved to Santa Fe and left their well-established classes to me. Their relocation coincided with my first retreat at the Last Resort. Filled with inspiration from a week of living a yogic life, I began teaching upon my return from the retreat.

In 1988 I attended my first vipassana retreat at the Last Resort. Since then I have attended a dozen more, each one infusing me with inspiration and opening me to new insight. Each meditation retreat, as well as so many life experiences that have followed, has called me ever more compellingly to my destiny.

I feel blessed to have met these incredible teachers who embody wisdom, compassion, and impeccable integrity. From Pujari and Abhilasha I have learned what it is to be a teacher. Above all, they have taught me that a student's path is unequivocally her own. Never in my years under their mentorship have they ever told me what my path is, where it should lead, or how I should walk it. Rather, they have taught me how to illuminate the trail so that I could—if I chose—see the treasures that reveal themselves when I pay attention. They have trusted me enough to let me fall, sometimes hard, knowing there was no other way for me to understand what it is to have fallen and to learn how to pick myself up.

Did they ever push my buttons? Absolutely. At times when I was not ready to let go of something that was causing pain, I avoided contact. I knew that the light of truth would shine ruthlessly on whatever was out of integrity in my life, but sometimes I just didn't want to see. Sometimes I needed to let things become intolerable before I could change.

Pujari and Abhilasha have offered all they know freely and without expectation. Some of what they shared has not yet become integrated within me. Other offerings illuminated with laser-beam precision the exact corner of my psyche where ignorance had previously rendered me blind.

I have learned that the process of awakening is a series of small steps, many of which seem inconsequential. The process has at times been maddeningly tedious. The summit cannot be reached, however, if a hiker tries to skip even one of the steps leading to it. It was not until I had gained the benefit of hindsight that I could see just how perfectly each step fit into the entire tableau. This journey continues.

Pujari and Abhilasha have shared in my darkest days and my greatest illuminations. They have taught me that darkness and illumination cannot exist independently of each other. Their commitment to truth inspires me to require nothing less than total authenticity from myself.

I have been fortunate to be guided by other teachers of great integrity as well. In particular, my work with Donna Farhi shattered my previous framework of understanding in the field of hatha yoga. Until 1993 I had understood the body as a mechanism that could be made perfect simply by following a neat and predictable series of adjustments. Exploring Donna's work freed me to experience the body-mind as a fluid, unpredictable, organic whole. I learned to see myself and everyone else as a question waiting to be explored, rather than clinging to the false security of formulaic instructions. Donna's commitment to her own continuing process of awakening is an inspiration. In our many years of friendship, she has become a cherished spiritual ally.

In 1989 I had the privilege of attending a three-week intensive at the Ramamani Iyengar Memorial Institute in Pune, India. There I learned volumes about all aspects of practice during daily asana and pranayama classes with Geeta and B. K. S. Iyengar. Practicing in India, the millennia-old seat of yoga, and immersing myself in the country's unique rhythm, expanded my understanding of yoga on a profound level.

The yogis who attend my classes continue to teach me. My greatest joy as a teacher occurs when students experience insights that I had never considered or that run counter to my own understanding. This is when I know the students have made the practice their own.

It is my wish that what follows will inspire committed yogis to strike out on their own trail, to seek their unique truth. My intention is not to blaze a trail that others may follow, because my trail will never be a perfect fit for anyone else. Rather, my intention is to present ideas that might inspire further investigation. I hope that my words can help switch on the light of wisdom and compassion that shines within and connects us all.

I offer my story as an example of the trajectory of one person's path. You may find it helpful for reflecting on your own story. What was your original call to awakening? Was it a specific event, or can you cite a series of experiences that have inspired you to look more deeply? What were the heavenly messengers that inspired you to seek a new way of being? How has your call to destiny affected your worldly and your spiritual life? Are the two really different?

When we reflect on the spark that began our endeavor to awaken, we reconnect with the original spirit that brought us to practice in the first place. This can bring renewed inspiration. When our path takes unpredictable or confusing turns, remembering our call to destiny and our subsequent journey can help us see how each step, each stumbling block, has brought us to our current place of understanding.

One essential insight that came from my original call to destiny at age thirteen has guided my life since then. It is this: If my own happiness is my responsibility, the same is true for everyone else. This helped me to see that there are many truths, as many as there are beings in the universe. While the understanding I gained during my sleepless night in 1968 was right for me, many people continue to find inspiration in other formal spiritual systems, most of which espouse philosophies that are radically different from mine. Other seekers find truth while treading a path entirely outside the structure of organized religion. All paths are right. All paths are sacred. Ultimately each person finds truth in a way that is congruous with his or her own integrity.

This insight underlies my philosophy for teaching yoga. For this reason I have chosen not to label my yogic style. I do not want to confine its evolution by naming it. More important, I want my students to find their own yoga, because I know that ultimately whatever I offer as a teacher must be understood and integrated within the context of each person's life. Labeling my style would make it too easy for my students to attribute whatever they have learned in their practice to my methods, and this would simply not be true. Whatever I have to offer as a teacher is given so that it may be the springboard to individual inquiry. I offer the ideas in this book in the same spirit, as a starting point for the exploration of your own truth.

So take time to reflect on your own personal journey and how you have come to be the person you are today. What personal philosophies have evolved through your practice? How do these philosophies guide your life? If you practice yoga, how has your practice altered your life? Listen deeply to the answers you hear when you ask these questions. They will help you clarify the path that lies ahead.

During a private consultation on a meditation retreat in 2003, Pujari presented me with a gift: He gave me the cedar walking stick he had used on his trek across America. The stick represents the courage, commitment, and determination it took for him to take each single step, thousands of which brought him to the end of that journey. The stick sits by my desk as I write. It guides each word. It radiates integrity. It inspires. It reminds me of all the steps it took for me to come to this place of beginning again.

Part I:

What Is Yoga?

Yoga: The Settling of the Mind 1

M Y CHILDHOOD HOME sits at the end of a dead-end street in the rolling hills of southeastern Indiana. Below the house are three acres of unruly woods that end abruptly at the edge of Hogan Creek, a tributary large enough to accommodate the recreational fancies of houseboat enthusiasts, water skiers and, in the wintertime, ice skaters. My favorite time of day there was evening. I loved sitting alone on the front step of our house watching the blackening sky, listening to cricket song, and watching the lazy-flashing lightning bugs punctuating the darkness. Most of all, I loved the silence. Inside the house, activity ruled—conversation, the tones of flute, clarinet, and piano, television. Outside there was only stillness and the deep blue-black sky sprinkled with starlight. Gazing at the sky, I felt its vastness. Stillness enveloped me, and I became peace.

Silence is what kept me tethered to Utah in my early years here. On my first trip to Arches National Park in April of 1983, I experienced true silence for the first time. In the early 1980s the park was relatively empty in springtime. This particular night there were only three or four other tents in the campground, pitched more than a hundred yards from my own. As daylight faded, I sat alone on a picnic table. In the desert landscape of southeastern Utah, no leaves rustle, no crickets sing. There was no wind this night. The silence was absolute, deafening. When a raven flew about fifty feet overhead, I heard the rhythmic whooshing of its wings. Ecstasy flooded my cells, enlivening me. I knew then that Utah was my home. I did not want to venture too far away from this incomparable resource, the austere, silent beauty of the desert.

When I began practicing yoga asana in 1982, it was the stillness of mind I felt that first captured me. I enjoyed the increased flexibility and freedom from back pain that I noticed soon after beginning practice, but most of all it was sense of pervading peace that drew me to commit to yoga. Although I was aware that asana practice was embedded in a larger philosophy, I chose not to learn about it until much later. The benefits I was feeling at the time were enough.

In the late 1990s, yoga asana (the practice of postures) became wildly popular in the West. What we call yoga in Western culture is more accurately termed asana. Yoga is much larger, encompassing all areas of our lives. Asana is one small part of the practice. Of the nearly two hundred Yoga Sutras, only three are concerned with asana. The purpose of asana is to prepare the body for meditation, which sutra scholar Alistair Shearer calls "the heart of yoga." The physical practices are designed to refine the body, specifically the nervous system. Because asana practice has always been integrated into the schedule at Last Resort meditation retreats, I was able to see firsthand how this works. In the context of consistent mindfulness practice, asana is truly a joy. Careful attention allowed me to drop beneath the level of gross sensation so I could experience and enjoy the subtle movements and energies in my body. Because asana unwinds musculoskeletal knots and promotes deep breathing, the practice makes sitting meditation much more comfortable. After asana practice, the body feels light and clear, the mind calm.

As a companion to meditation practice, I have maintained an interest in the concepts presented in the Abhidhamma, the comprehensive text on Buddhist psychology. I learned what I knew of Buddhist philosophy by reading books by such wise and insightful teachers as Joseph Goldstein, Sharon Salzberg, Jack Kornfield, and Thich Nhat Hanh, and through hearing hundreds of taped dharma talks by these and other Western teachers. These distillations of the teachings resonated profoundly with my understanding and my life.

What I did not realize was how many parallels existed between what I had learned through Buddhist channels and the wisdom crystallized in the Yoga Sutras. When I decided to embark on a reading of the Yoga Sutras, I found that much of what I already understood through meditation practice was written there. For this reason, I weave the two philosophies together throughout this text.

Around 300 B.C.E., a sage named Patanjali codified the ancient wisdom that is yoga. While the ideas presented in the sutras are likely a composite of timeless, universal wisdom that had evolved over the ages, Patanjali brought the concepts together into a definitive text that serves as a succinct, almost step-by-step map of the inner journey of awakening. Written in Sanskrit, the aphorisms are short, concise, and devoid of any literary coloration. Sanskrit does not accurately translate word-for-word to English, so translators have added their own interpretations to the text. Many Sanskrit words symbolize concepts that do not have direct English correlations. For this reason, I've found it most helpful to use multiple translations in my own sutra study. Each different translation adds dimension to the meaning of each verse.

The entire volume of sutras is crystallized in the second aphorism. All subsequent sutras aim to define and explain the concept and introduce all the methods of practice that lead to the state of yoga. Many years before setting my intention to study the sutras, a teaching colleague repeated a translation of this single, defining verse. At that time, the translation seemed abstract and somewhat forceful to me, and initially it turned me away from pursuing yogic philosophy. Of course, this was rather shortsighted, but my interest had not reached the critical mass necessary to inspire me to take a closer look. Who knew there was more than one way of interpreting a sutra?

Patanjali's second aphorism gives the definition of yoga, as it was explained to me at that time: "Yoga is the stopping of the fluctuations in the mind." From my meditation experience, I understood very well what those fluctuations were. I had met and become endlessly annoyed with the "wild monkey," the traditional Buddhist metaphor for the untrained mind. Somehow the cessation of the monkey's taunts seemed far, far away, if not impossible. It also seemed tantamount to clamping my consciousness down entirely. Later I would discover that while this was quite close to being an exact literal translation, other interpretations would help me understand and appreciate this sutra more fully.

The original Sanskrit for the second sutra is *yogas citta vrtti nirodah*. In his scholarly volume *The Yoga Sutra of Patanjali*, Georg Feuerstein translates each word literally from the Sanskrit: *yogas* = yoga, *citta* = consciousness, *vrtti* = fluctuation, *nirodah* = restriction. Based on his direct word-for-word translation, Feuerstein's interpretation of the aphorism reads, "Yoga is the restriction of the fluctuations of consciousness." This translation, which is remarkably similar to the first translation I heard many years before, became my ground for exploring this sutra. Subtle differences in wording—"restriction" versus "stopping," "consciousness" versus "mind," even "of" instead of "in"—gave my original understanding greater dimension. Still, I sought a translation that did not imply what I interpreted as a closing down of mind.

Barbara Stoler Miller, author of *Yoga: Discipline of Freedom*, offers this translation: "Yoga is the cessation of the turnings of thought." The word "cessation" gives a sense of greater ease to the sutra. In this translation, there is an implication that mental fluctuations can stop naturally without the imposition of force. The venerable T. K. V. Desikachar's translation, from his book *Patanjali's Yogasutras*, fleshes out the concept further. His take on the sutra is "Yoga is the ability to direct the mind exclusively towards an object and sustain that direction without any distractions." Directing and sustaining the mind implies an active movement in a specific direction. Perhaps this is what causes the cessation of mental fluctuations. Because each translation reflects the author's personal experience, I always consider many translations in my sutra study. A single translator's ideas do not always paint a complete picture.

Alistair Shearer offers the translation of this sutra that best suits my current understanding. While not literal, this poetic interpretation distills the meaning of yoga in a way that fits with my personal experience. Shearer translates Sutra I.2: "Yoga is the settling of the mind into silence."

I love this translation on many levels. First is its overall positive nature. In this interpretation, yoga is achieved not by stopping something but by a gentle, incremental process of release. I love the word "settling." To settle implies relaxation into a state that is natural and inherent; it is a verb that suggests a process. It implies a gradual, continuous release, rather than the reaching of a static endpoint. Shearer's translation does not tell us to look outside ourselves to find stillness and peace. That silence is something we can settle into more deeply with each breath. The stillness is who we are, not something we must attain.

What is this stillness? We can touch stillness by visiting nature. Taking a walk in silence with occasional stops to enjoy whatever is present in the environment—the sights, the sounds, the feel of the earth beneath us, the feel of the atmosphere, the wind and sun on our skin—helps to ground the mind in stillness. The desert is the epitome of stillness. A lake, glassy still on a windless day, teaches us about silence. But sometimes even the quiet of the desert is disturbed. A silent lake is easily agitated by rain, wind, and wildlife. Where is a reliable source of stillness to be found?

Stillness resides in awareness. My favorite metaphor for awareness is the sky—clear and infinite. No matter what disturbances appear in the sky, the sky itself remains unchanged. Clouds may pass through. Thunderstorms create temporary turbulence. Winds stir up the atmosphere. Air pollution muddies our view. Light pollution obscures the stars. Yet the sky itself is not tarnished by these events. It remains vast, pure, impartial.

Awareness is exactly the same. Awareness is the quality inherent to all of us; it can experience the careening of the wild monkey mind with its emotional peaks and valleys, its agitations, and its illuminations, without relinquishing its essential purity. Awareness is vast and limitless, clear and luminous. Donna Farhi describes awareness in her book *Bringing Yoga to Life* as a screen onto which all our experience is projected. The screen is not the same as what is projected upon it. It simply reflects. This impartial screen is the core stillness that lives within each of us. It envelops and binds us all. The practice of yoga in all its aspects allows us to reconnect with and dwell in awareness, our essential being.

My first five-day vipassana meditation retreat in 1988 was not a sterling example of the settled mind. I could not have previously imagined the pure frustration of the first three days, which were hellish beyond anything I had experienced in my life up to that point. My knees ached, my lower back screamed, my left shoulder felt as if it was being stabbed continuously. But the physical discomfort I felt was no match for the mental torment. A riot of rampant thoughts, ranging from ridiculous to annoying to downright enraging, charged through my mind at all times. Among the most prominent assaults were mental whining about the physical pain, serious doubts about the worth of the practice and the abilities of my teachers, and a pervasive desire to be anywhere but sitting on that unforgiving hardwood bench. A parade of long-forgotten annoying songs and catchy commercial jingles from the '60s provided cruel background music for it all. Nonstop mental carping soured the entire mix.

The instructions that were given were to watch the breath, either the sensation of the breath entering and leaving the nostrils or the sensation of the rising and falling of the abdomen. My mind was everywhere but on the breath. Even keeping my mind focused on a single inhalation was too much to ask. I felt endlessly frustrated and angry at myself for failing so miserably at something that should have been pretty simple. Walking meditation was only slightly less discouraging. Paying attention to the mechanics of each plodding step at least gave me somewhere a bit less subtle to aim my mind. Still, wild, erratic thought dominated my experience in walking meditation as well.

Much of my abundant mental energy was occupied with constructing elaborate fantasies about how I might bow out gracefully. I could walk down to the public phone a half-mile away, call my husband, and have him come pick me up in the middle of the night while everyone was sleeping. I would simply disappear. When I was having a particularly bad time, I would throw the idea of grace out the window and fantasize about jumping up off the relentlessly hard meditation bench and running out of the room screaming.

Still, I resentfully persevered. On the third day, I was preparing to brush my teeth before retiring—ah, sleep, that lovely time of day when I escaped the continuous barrage of mental refuse. As I reached for the bathroom doorknob, I continued practice. I paid close attention to the subtle sensation of my extending elbow joint and bicep muscles; the cool, surprising smoothness of the knob; the rotation of the bones in my forearm as I turned the knob. The experience was absolutely exquisite. After opening thousands of doors in my life, this was the first time I had felt what it is to turn a doorknob.

This simple moment of experiencing the fullness of the present moment turned my practice around. My body still ached and my mind still ran out of control most of the time, but now I knew why I was practicing. That timeless moment of mindfulness had shown me the richness and satisfaction of living in the present. The desire to embody mindfulness had been awakened. It has never left.

At breakfast the next day, the crunchy explosion of textures and flavors in my morning granola was almost too much sensation for me to assimilate. I practiced asana that morning with renewed curiosity and attention to the subtlest movements. Poses I had done hundreds of times felt completely new and delicious. For much of the day, I felt a sense of joy so intense and absolute that I thought (quite mistakenly) that I must be enlightened. Colors were more vibrant, my eyesight more crystalline. I became absorbed in sounds that would have been irritating the previous day. Later that afternoon my mind settled into a pervading peace like none I had ever experienced. I sat easily without moving for an entire one-hour period, a feat that I could not have imagined just a day earlier.

In the evening my practice shifted back into its usual chaos. The aching in my knees intensified, and my mind went back to its endless chattering. I longed for the peace and joy I had felt just hours earlier. I surmised from my apparent backslide that I was indeed not enlightened, as I had previously thought. I also learned about a very important truth: everything changes.

That all things are impermanent is the core of the Buddha's teaching. The first of his four noble truths, that life is suffering, is based on the understanding that, because everything changes, there is nothing we can rely upon as being a permanent source of happiness. Furthermore, there is nothing in our experience that we can hold on to long enough to fashion a permanent "self," although we certainly try. The understanding of impermanence is essential to living in freedom. When we stop chasing happiness in the form of material goods, experiences, and relationships that, because of their impermanent nature, will never ultimately satisfy us, we open ourselves to the possibility of uncovering the lasting happiness that dwells within—the settled mind.

I do not know of a more direct way to experience the truth of impermanence than to sit quietly and mindfully watch whatever phenomena pass through my consciousness. Had I not been overcome by my identification with frustration early in my first retreat, I could have seen this rather easily even then. Viewed with microscopic attention, the stabbing in my shoulder was not the solid, constant barrage of pain I had thought it to be. In reality the sensation of pain was present only some of the time. Every few seconds it would arise, intensify, and then retreat. Each occurrence was slightly different from the previous one.

At that time I was not yet ready to see my experience of constantly shifting physical pain as an indication of a progressively strengthening practice. Rather, I thought that the presence of pain was an indication that I was doing something wrong—giving me one more reason to pass judgment on my practice. But my understanding here was unclear, muddied by my preferences. In the same way that I felt each incremental movement as I reached for the doorknob, I had begun to awaken to the changing sensations of my various aches and pains. It would take a few more days of resisting discomfort for me to understand that even physical pain can be a door to insight.

Because the doorknob experience was in the pleasurable realm, I was willing to recognize it as an experience of some level of absorption. In that simple act, all that existed for me were the ever-changing sensations of reaching, touching, and turning. In essence I became the process of reaching, touching, and turning in that moment. There was an instant knowing of each momentary sensation, yet I was not engaging in any sort of thinking process. Without the filter of thought evaluating each sensation, the experience was intimate beyond my imagining.

No matter how many thousands of times I had turned a doorknob during my lifetime, I saw in this moment that this experience, right now, is totally new. I did not turn the knob any differently than I ever had, nor was it an extraordinary doorknob. The external conditions were irrelevant. What made it exquisite was the level of presence I brought to the process.

In his book *The Miracle of Mindfulness*, Thich Nhat Hanh writes about "washing the dishes to wash the dishes." Instead of washing the dishes in order to get to the cup of tea you will have afterward, he encourages us to engage fully in the act of washing the dishes. Viewed with careful attention, the experience of dishwashing yields a surprising richness of sensation—the feeling of warm, sudsy water, the smoothness and weight of the plates in your hands, the movements of scrubbing and rinsing. Any activity can become a wondrous and sacred ritual if we pay attention.

The book's chapter titled "The Miracle Is to Walk on Earth" describes mindful walking along a path into a village. Nhat Hanh writes, "You practice by keeping this one thought alive: 'I'm walking along the path leading into the village.' Whether it's sunny or rainy, whether the path is dry or wet, you keep that one thought, but not just repeating it like a machine, over and over again. Machine thinking is the opposite of mindfulness. If we're really engaged in mindfulness while walking along the path to the village, then we will consider the act of each step we take as an infinite wonder, and a joy will open our hearts like a flower, enabling us to enter the world of reality."

Mindfulness is the thread that connects all aspects of yoga practice. When we give our full attention to what we are doing, we become that which is present in our experience. If I am mindful, when I teach yoga, I am simply and completely a yoga teacher; when I play music, I am an oboist; when I wash dishes, I am a dishwasher; when I practice asana, I become the asana; when I eat, I am a diner; when I walk, I am a walker. When I engage mindfully in even the most trivial of my life's activities, my life is full and satisfying no matter what I am doing. When we live our lives mindfully, we live in fullness; there is no leftover residue of regret for missed opportunities.

Mindfulness is most commonly practiced in sitting and walking meditation. If you can sit quietly for even a few minutes each day, watching the flow of your breath, you will begin to strengthen the power of your mind. But mindfulness practice needn't be confined to formal meditation. Every activity in which you engage throughout your day provides an opportunity to be mindful.

You might begin the practice of mindful living by choosing one activity, something you do each day, where you will be completely present. Washing the dishes, cooking, enjoying a cup of tea, brushing your teeth, driving to work, showering, practicing an instrument, taking a walk—the activity you choose does not matter as much as the care and respect you bring to it. Being mindful of something you are already doing does not require that you make space in your schedule for something new. You're already washing the dishes. Why not pay attention?

You could begin your practice with your morning tea. Pay careful attention as you fill the teakettle. Feel the handle of the teakettle vibrating as water pours in. Note the sensation of contact when you place the teakettle on the burner. Feel the rotation of your wrist as you turn on the burner. Listen to the gradual intensity of sound as the water begins to boil. Feel the weight of the teakettle in your hand, and how the weight shifts as the water pours into the cup. Feel the altered weight of the pot and the sloshing movement of the water inside as you set it down. As you prepare to drink, feel your arm gliding through the air as you reach for the cup. How does the heated smoothness of the cup feel in your hand? What is the sensation of lifting the cup? How does the lip of the cup feel against your own? What is the feeling of hot liquid as it reaches your tongue and slides down your throat? What is the sensation of taste? How does the taste evolve? Drinking a cup of tea, washing the dishes, or even emptying the litter box can be at the very least engaging, and possibly profoundly satisfying, if we bring ourselves fully to the activity.

Drinking a cup of tea mindfully in the quiet of the morning is one of the sublime pleasures of my life. While I drink my tea I leave the newspaper folded. I do not unzip my day planner until after I've finished. I enjoy every moment of the tea ceremony, from the heating of the kettle to the last sip. I like to think that the thread of mindfulness begun at tea then weaves its way throughout other parts of my day.

Often when I've felt bored or disengaged from what I'm doing, I have found that raising my level of attention generates energy and interest. This leads me to wonder if boredom is simply a symptom of an underlying lack of attention. When we meet even the most seemingly pedestrian experiences with a sense of interest and care, they can become fascinating.

The key here is to remember that there is no time but the present. What is past exists only in thought. Author and meditation teacher Joseph Goldstein has likened dwelling in reveries or regrets about the past to lugging around a corpse. How many times do we have to recount the details of some past hurt and make ourselves feel bad about it? On the other hand, future thinking is truly fantasy. We really don't know what's going to happen next, yet so much mental energy is invested in speculation, planning, and worry about the future.

Worry happens to be one of my special habits. A manifestation of restlessness, worry has kept me awake many nights. The interesting thing is, most of the time the things I worry about never happen. There is a Zen story about a cave-dwelling monk who paints a very realistic picture of a tiger and then looks at it and gets scared. This is exactly what we do when we worry. We make up a story of what we think will happen, and then we fret about it. I've heard the Dalai Lama quoted as saying, "If there is a solution to a problem, there is no need to worry. And if there is no solution, there is no need to worry."

The other prevalent type of future thinking has to do with desire. We imagine that somehow the future will be better than right now. But it is only in the present moment that we can be truly satisfied. When we are engaged in whatever is occurring right now, there is no room for desire or worry. The mind can settle only when the agitations of thought are not pulling it hither and yon. Our lives are happening here and now. Don't miss your life by dwelling in the past or future!

Reflections

- Choose to be mindful of something you do each day. It can be something you enjoy doing or something you don't especially like. You might want to choose one of each. Over time, notice how your relationship to these daily tasks begins to shift. I love this practice because it shows us how to apply a simple meditative technique to the way we live.

The Flowering of Mindfulness 2

MY VEGETABLE GARDEN is conceived each year in the gray days of February. As the delicate, resolute crocus shoots poke through the frozen earth in my front yard, my intention turns to the annual ritual of turning soil in my backyard. As soon as the snow has melted from my garden plots, I begin testing the ground. When the soil is dry enough to turn without sliding off my shovel in huge, soggy clumps (and breaking my back from its heft), I begin softening the beds. I break up the soil into loosely packed, fine grains that will easily give way to delicate emerging seedlings.

I nourish the soil by working in rich organic compost. As seedlings emerge, I spend time each week uprooting the tenacious weeds that compete for their nutrients. A drip system waters each plant. In April, when the plants are still tiny, it is hard to imagine the overabundance of produce I will likely enjoy by August. Yet, after so many years of repeating and refining this process, I have learned to trust that when I give care and attention to each step, my garden flourishes, often in ways I could not have imagined. Some years the leafy greens are most prolific and tasty; other years the tomato plants tower over me, yielding an amazing abundance of fruit.

What I love about gardening is not only the process of working the soil and planting the seeds but also seeing my efforts take form. The results are both predictable—I literally reap what I sow—and unpredictable: who would have thought that a single vine could hold seventy tomatoes?

While the garden may be the most literal way to observe the planting of seeds and reaping of fruit, there are countless other examples in our lives.

When a pianist practices scales, her fingers become more facile. When the same pianist practices the music she loves, her playing becomes more lyrical and heartfelt. With time and dedication, a runner's stamina increases, her heart rate slows, and she becomes more energetic and clear-headed. A person who loves to read becomes a more skilled reader and often becomes a more creative writer or speaker, simply from immersing herself in artful language.

Practicing mindfulness, too, bears both predictable and unpredictable fruits. The most immediately palpable benefit of mindfulness practice is that of simple awareness—the careful, microscopic attention that, when brought to daily tasks, can render them satisfying and even fascinating. Awareness, the silent screen that reflects all our experiences, is the process through which we discover the settled mind and is the settled mind itself. It is both the means and the end. From the cultivation of awareness grows deeper awareness. Its flowers bear the seeds of still other nourishing fruits.

To commemorate the twentieth anniversary of beginning his vipassana practice, insight meditation teacher Steven Armstrong gave a talk to people attending a three-month meditation retreat at Insight Meditation Society in November of 1995. In the talk he listed what he had found to be the five beautiful qualities that develop from living a mindful life—awareness, authenticity, caring, contentment, and creativity.

I've observed the blossoming of these qualities in my friends in the dharma community and have watched them evolve through my own practice. But until I heard Armstrong's talk, it had never occurred to me that they are a natural, and likely a universal, result of committed practice. Outlining the benefits of mindfulness in this way not only confirms my observations but also clarifies the fruits of meditation practice in a way that inspires even greater commitment.

Awareness

Awareness is the first of the beautiful attributes that develops from mindful living. It is the fertile ground from which all the other qualities flourish. When we are paying attention, our minds are at peace, not being pulled hither and yon by reactions to thoughts and emotions. Thought and emotion may well be present, but we feel them fully and observe them in process, rather than being overcome by them.

The first time I looked closely at my mind, I was astonished to see how completely out of control it really was. Like the wild monkey of Buddhist metaphor, my mind careened from elation and excitement to anger and despair, depending on the thoughts present at the time. What was even more astonishing was how repetitive my thoughts were, and how often I energized myself by focusing on thoughts that upset me, thoughts that usually fell into the category of worrying about something that may or may not ever happen.

Now I understand the futility of worry, but it took many years for me to uproot this deeply cultivated conditioning. One of the great gifts of mindfulness is that it reveals what mental habits dominate us and, more important, gives us the choice to continue to feed them or not.

Thought patterns fall into one of two categories: reminiscences of the past and fantasies about the future. When we are caught in either scenario, we are not connected with what is present and true in this moment. Thinking itself is not a problem. The problem lies in how we relate to our thoughts. Quite often we are lost in the story unfolding in our thoughts, usually reacting emotionally in some way. How many times do we need to replay the ancient tale of someone treating us badly in the past? How many times do we want to reinforce the anger and hurt we felt in response? How often do we react emotionally to thoughts about something we are worried will happen that may not ever take place? These are ways we confuse and agitate our minds. It is possible instead to be present with the process of thinking. We can be aware that thinking is occurring without getting lost in the content of our thoughts.

This is not to say that mindful reflection on our past actions is not sometimes helpful. It is one of the ways we learn from our missteps and our successes. But there is a difference between conscious reflection that results in a resolve to act more skillfully in the future and tormenting ourselves by dredging up memories of our regretful actions and then punishing ourselves again and again.

When we turn our minds toward what is present right now, we find rest. We cannot be fully mindful and distracted by thought simultaneously. In simply watching the arising and passing of thought and sensation, without grasping or pushing them away, we can dwell in peaceful awareness. In awareness we are balanced in the fluid movement of the ever-changing present moment. Awareness is the settled mind, which sees clearly, directly, and impartially what is true, unclouded by conditioning and opinions.

Authenticity

The word *vipassana* means "clear seeing." A few years into my practice, I had what might seem like a very obvious insight. As I sat in meditation, watching the parade of physical, mental, and emotional events arise and pass, it occurred to me that in each mind moment of pure awareness, I was experiencing a direct encounter with Truth. A huge wave of gratitude flooded my cells. I felt honored that I had managed to stumble upon this practice. The simplicity and directness of vipassana meditation felt nothing short of sublime: Pay attention. That's all. So simple, so miraculous.

In that moment, whatever sensations happened to be arising were inconsequential compared to the knowing of them. In retrospect, the insight was the embodiment of a concept I had considered intellectually many times, but this was different. It had entered the level of deep, cellular knowing, and I was instantly, irrevocably changed. I had had an encounter with truth, that same truth that is available to us all in each moment of awareness. This time, however, I knew it.

It is the quality of knowing that distinguishes mindfulness as a form of meditation. And it is the deep knowing of our momentary experience that gives us access to our innermost desires and fears. In the process of seeing, accepting, and letting go of our experience as it arises and passes, we begin to peel away layers of conditioned thought and behavior patterns based on desire and fear. No longer blinded by the filters of conditioning, we see more clearly what is actually present.

This deep level of knowing allows us to act from our most profound truth. In the process of settling into deeper awareness of ourselves, we move ever closer to the core of who we are. As we identify and begin the process of shedding those patterns that obscure our clear seeing, we begin to live with greater authenticity. The center of our own truth becomes our reference point. It becomes more difficult to act in opposition to what we know to be true. "Walking our talk" becomes a habit. Choices are immediately clear, because we understand our intentions and feel the rightness or wrongness of a choice as we contemplate it. As we approach our deepest integrity, our intentions and actions become more aligned with what will serve the greater good. It becomes difficult to act outside our integrity.

As I have become more aware of my own authentic center, I have had to let go of certain habits and relationships because I could no longer deny that they had become inappropriate. This is one of the perils of spiritual practice. It is also one of its great gifts. Sometimes we must move on, letting go of situations that have been dear to us. It is helpful to reflect on the many things that were once precious to you that you have released from your life. There are countless examples, from childhood games to adolescent angst, from high school sweethearts to that first job at the burger joint. What became available to you when you let go of a habit or relationship that was truly finished?

Mindfulness is the key to finding your own authentic yoga practice and allowing that practice to grow and blossom. Early in my asana practice, I focused on perfecting the form of the yoga asanas and learning the more advanced positions. As time has passed, I find a slow, meditative practice to be much more profound, and more powerful. What I have released in terms of attention to the more outward manifestations of asana practice, I have gained in terms of subtle awareness, steadiness, and inner strength. Mindfulness has given me the trust to allow my practice to change in hundreds of ways over the years. As I have tested for myself what I have read and learned from others about yoga, and learned to trust my direct observations, my practice has become my own. When I am mindful, I can easily let go of ideas about yoga that do not fit, making room for new ways of seeing and practicing. When I am connected with my own authentic center, I can flow easily with the evolution of my practice and my life.

Caring

Retreats at the Last Resort are small and intimate. Participants eat, sleep, sit, and practice asana in Pujari and Abhilasha's house. The combination of physical closeness and the settling of minds engenders a profound respect and caring for the cocoon of quiet woven through days and weeks of practice. Participants become sensitive to harsh energies. When I am on retreat, I tread lightly through the cabin. I open and close doors with care. I consider how my attitudes and actions might affect those around me.

Vipassana retreats are traditionally held in silence. On retreats at the Last Resort, as well as at other centers I've visited, we maintain silence not just because it is the agreement we have made at the outset of the retreat. We refrain from speaking because of a sense of caring for the precious silent space. We hold that space as one would a tiny kitten, with great attention and gentleness.

Caring for the well-being of others is a manifestation of the understanding that we are all interconnected. Our actions, for good or for ill, do affect those around us. Our kind words have an uplifting effect, and our harsh words cause the other to shrink away. Words spoken mindlessly can confuse or cause hurt. Caring arises from the empathy cultivated in mindfulness practice. When we see clearly and directly into our own capacity for joy and sorrow, we understand that everyone has these same capacities.

The sense of caring cultivated on retreat reminds me to respect the time and energy of those around me. Deep caring also reaches into my relationship with my environment. I walk more gently on the earth, being conscious of my use of resources—the air, water, and land that belong to all of us.

Taken a step further, caring can manifest as the desire to share our time, energy, skills, and resources for the benefit of others. Mindfulness connects us with our most basic desire—to be happy. As awareness deepens, we begin to understand that all beings share this desire. We realize that the happiness of others is no different from our own. From this understanding, we are compelled to offer our gifts freely. In his talk on the beautiful qualities of mindful living, Steven Armstrong said, "Give what and to whom makes you happy."

Contentment

The vipassana retreat routine is relentless. Each day's schedule is the same: sit, walk, sit, yoga, breakfast, walk, sit, walk, sit—on and on throughout the day, from 5:30 in the morning until 9:30 at night. In a sense, the routine is quite freeing. The mind is not bothered with decisions. There are few surprises. Over days and weeks of practice, however, it is easy to observe the daily plateaus and valleys in our inner realms of existence. The schedule's stark monotony shows us unequivocally that happiness and unhappiness have little to do with external conditions.

This understanding first dawned on me at the end of a two-day period filled with extreme highs and lows—elation followed by frustration followed by calm followed by chaos. As I reflected on the preceding days' experiences, I realized that while my mind had taken extraordinary journeys, through peaks and valleys and all that lies between, nothing had changed outwardly. On both days I was surrounded by crystalline high desert beauty. I sat, walked, practiced asana, and took my meals with the same people. The food was fantastic—delicious and lovingly prepared. The dharma talks were superb. Given the relative pleasantness of retreat, what caused my mind to swing to and fro, from happiness to unhappiness and back, so many times each day?

Living in such ideal conditions for practice, it was easy to see that my inner drama had nothing to do with my surroundings. It had everything to do with my willingness or unwillingness to accept what was present in each moment's experience. Seeing the power of my responses to dictate my mental and emotional well-being, I was compelled to relax. In that relaxation, I discovered contentment.

Contentment is a sense of deep satisfaction with life as it is. It is born of the understanding that all things arise and pass according to natural law. We gain this insight by giving careful attention to whatever arises in each moment. In practicing acceptance of all that arises and passes within our mental landscape, we cultivate the ability to be at peace with our present predicament.

Smiling—or more likely, gritting your teeth—and barely tolerating your life is not contentment. Rather, contentment is the acceptance of and gratitude for the gift of your life as it is, with all its peaks and valleys, which give you the vital opportunity to learn about yourself.

The cultivation of contentment is one of the niyamas, or observances, and one branch of the second limb in Patanjali's eight-limbed path of yoga. We will revisit the cultivation of contentment when we explore the traditional system of yoga in chapter 14.

Creativity

I first discovered that I enjoyed writing in fifth grade, when my friend Chandra and I wrote animal stories—mostly about cats and horses—for fun. As a teenager I enjoyed writing essays and op-ed pieces for the school paper. Throughout my college career, as I was experimenting with mind-altering chemicals, which promised to open my mind to unexplored creative possibilities, my writing life became a barren desert. On the rare occasion when I was able to squeeze out a three-page paper, I always saved it for future reuse. My greatest challenge was remembering which professors had already seen the paper and making sure I didn't submit it to the same one twice.

During this time, much of my inner world was a mystery, a dusty book I preferred to open as little as possible. My chemical habits brought me out of my more comfortable state of introversion. What I sacrificed in inner awareness, I gained in social education, which ultimately brought me to greater fullness as a worldly human being. I was content with this trade-off. Still, each time I pulled out a worn-out paper to submit a second or third time, I wondered what had happened to my former love of writing.

Assuming my early forays into writing had been just a phase, I gave the subject little thought until I enrolled in school again, nine years after graduating with my bachelor's degree. When I learned that my basic writing course credits would not transfer from Indiana University to the University of Utah, a little gray cloud of dread settled in: I would have to retake the class. I wondered if I had any of those papers I wrote at Indiana. In the first week of the course I learned that we would be assigned weekly writing exercises. The little gray cloud turned dark and menacing.

This was early 1989, and I had just come home from a ten-day mindfulness retreat when I began taking university classes. Having spent more than a week clearing out my repetitive thought patterns, my mind was a clean slate compared to its usual chaotic jumble. Much to my great surprise and delight, the dreaded writing exercises were a joy from the moment I took up my pen. Ideas flowed faster than I could write them down. My long-lost love of writing had awakened from its fifteen-year hibernation.

I realized that the clearing of my mental slate was allowing new creative ideas to flow. The repetitive patterns that so annoy us in meditation practice leave no space in our mental environment for anything else to germinate. In the same way weeds in the garden crowd out the plants we want to cultivate, habitual thought patterns take root in our mental environment. They deplete the soil and spread their vines into the entire garden plot. Left untended, they seed themselves indefinitely.

When we weed out our persistent patterns, creative energy flourishes. Our lives become revitalized. Creativity is the ground of our life force. The reproductive energy that allows all life on earth to proliferate is creativity at its most elemental level. When we nurture our creativity, our lives are constantly renewed. When we are mindful, we become more available to the arising of creative energy. As we cease spending our vital energies on repetitive mental habits, those energies are released to us to use in a multitude of ways.

Sit awhile and watch the landscape in your mind. Can you identify repetitive, self-perpetuating thought loops that are going nowhere? Each time we give these patterns permission to run their course, and each time we identify with them, they wear deeper grooves in our psyches. These well-trodden trails become the paths of least resistance.

Ask yourself where you would like to spend your precious creative energy. If you like where the familiar thought patterns take you, you may choose to continue the relationship. If you find you'd like to infuse your life with more surprising energies and ideas, set the familiar aside. You will probably have to be persistent. Watch what appears.

Because yoga practice is really about how we live our lives, the opportunities to practice mindfulness and to manifest its beautiful attributes are many. The eight-limbed path of yoga encompasses all areas of life and practice. As you read about each limb, take it to heart and apply it to your life. Spread the seeds of mindfulness throughout all your daily practices—asana, meditation, household chores, work, and family. Watch your life flower.

Part II:

Refining Practice

.

The Path of Practice: 3
Making Practice Your Art

MUSIC WAS the ever-present anchor of my childhood. My parents met while taking lessons from the same vocal teacher. My two sisters and I began taking piano lessons at age eight and continued through high school and beyond. Later we each learned another instrument as well. Evenings in our household were cacophonous. Each room in the house embodied a unique sonic experience, sometimes pleasant, sometimes grating, as we explored our respective instruments. My parents must have developed a phenomenal tolerance for the sound of sour notes.

"Practice" was the word of the era. There was no compromising practice time. I often felt culturally deprived compared with my classmates. I was clueless about the latest primetime shows. By the time we finished homework and practice in the evening, it was time for bed. When my friends sang the theme songs to Saturday morning cartoons, I could not join in. I was never home on Saturday mornings, because this was when we made our weekly trek to Cincinnati for music lessons.

Early on, I wondered about the value of practicing tedious long tones on my oboe and the mechanical scales and arpeggios on both instruments. My youthful fingers were short and awkward. The process of making a sound by blowing into the tiny and very resistant oboe reed gave me head rushes. It was a whole lot of work, and the rewards were not apparent. What exactly was the point?

Gradually I began to notice a pleasing shift in my practice. Once in a while I would experience moments when I was actually making music. Instead of laboriously poring over exercises and etudes, concentrating on every note, effort dissolved and music flowed. At those times I was no longer in charge. When I had invested a piece with enough time, intention, and work, it entered my cells and spilled out onto the keys of our Steinway. Playing music increasingly became a joy.

I can't begin to count the times I heard that there is no substitute for practice. As much as I have wanted to resist the concept, it is undeniable. Continual practice of anything, from piano to pitching to painting, imprints our chosen disciplines into our very cells. After years of watching my mind in meditation, I realize that practice can also happen subconsciously, in the many mental patterns that I have accumulated over the years that now manifest automatically in my reactions to the events of daily life. I'm glad to have practiced some of these, and others I now practice to undo.

In 1982 asana became my chosen practice. I was shocked at how tightly bound my body was in the beginning. Practice wrought a whole range of unpleasant sensations—pulling, tension, trembling, dizziness, nausea. Still, at the end of each practice, after lying in the final relaxation pose, I felt an inner stillness I could not have previously imagined. That was the reason I continued.

As months and years passed, my body and mind became more facile. Gradually the great effort I had invested into learning the art of asana integrated itself into my being. Now, even when I experience difficulty, I appreciate the motivation to look more deeply. These are the moments of exploration and creativity, and they often lead to insight. As it had with music, the pleasure of practice became the reason to continue. But unlike my experience with music, I do not practice to polish my skills for some future performance. Practice is an end in itself.

I have committed more time and energy to the practice of mindfulness than any other discipline. In two decades of mindfulness practice, I have watched my mind evolve through many stages of facility. But this movement is not necessarily linear. My mind can move from its monkey nature to sublime states of peace and then back to the taunting ape with great facility. I've learned to accept these seeming backslides as part of the process. Evolution takes time and energy. I was a permissive parent with my wild monkey mind for almost thirty years. It is only natural for a mind unaccustomed to boundaries to rebel against discipline.

Many years ago my older sister introduced me to a four-stage model for learning that I have seen play itself out innumerable times in many areas of my life. It is based in variations on two concepts—consciousness and competence.

The first stage of any learning process is unconscious incompetence. At this time in the process, we are not yet versed enough in our endeavor to know that we are unskillful. At this first stage of mindfulness practice, wildly erratic thought streams run themselves beyond our control. Because we have long practiced living in the realm of thinking, it is this pattern that has become integrated in us. It is familiar and therefore feels comfortable, even when we are caught in thoughts that evoke afflictive, sometimes painful mental states. We are unconscious of this pattern because it has become second nature. We lack the competence to change it because we are unconscious.

The second stage of learning is conscious incompetence. Here we have set an intention to practice a skill but have not yet developed the faculties to accomplish it. In learning to play the piano, at this stage I became aware of the mistakes I was making while playing my scales. This stage requires heroic effort, as we watch ourselves making lots of missteps. We play our scales over and over again, breaking down each phrase to train our fingers to play the right notes. At this stage in meditation, I could see that my mind was running here and there, completely out of control, but I lacked the skills to change it. I caught myself lost in thoughts innumerable times, well after their stories had sucked me into a vortex of drama. But unlike the first stage of practice, I caught myself at least some of the time.

The development of wisdom is available to us at this stage. If we remain aware, in meditation we can identify the patterns that run our lives and decide which ones we want to cultivate and which ones we want to change. In the case of practicing an instrument, we can see clearly our strengths and weaknesses, and we can choose how to bolster our strengths and focus on developing those aspects that lack skill.

Committed practice brings us to the third stage, conscious competence. At this point, we can see when we falter, and we falter less often. We must still invest a lot of energy, but our skills are up to the task. A pianist in this stage is working through a piece. She is playing the right notes but still thinks about what she is doing. If she is preparing a piece for performance, she is reading the music, following its instructions quite literally, and thinking about how she will interpret phrasing and dynamics.

At this stage in meditation practice, we have developed the awareness to see easily when the mind is wandering and the skill to bring the mind continuously back to what is happening. There is still great effort required, but that effort is much more refined. We become adept at catching our minds earlier in their excursions. We have developed skills that are more nuanced. Vigilance is still necessary, but our skills are sufficient to accomplish what we intend.

The Yoga Sutras of Patanjali describe the fourth learning stage, unconscious competence, quite well. One of the volume's three aphorisms devoted to asana practice, Sutra II.47, defines mastery of asana. As translated by Alistair Shearer, the sutra says, "[Asana] is mastered when all effort is relaxed and the mind is absorbed in the Infinite." This sutra aptly describes the final stage of practice in any discipline. At this stage, the discipline has become so much a part of us that we no longer have to think about it. Our skills reside in our cells. This is where practice becomes poetry.

It was not until a recent weeklong meditation retreat that I consistently enjoyed this stage of practice. I had experienced it in earlier meditations, but it lasted only for short periods. This time, rather than continually corralling my mind back to the present, I was able to rest in awareness of my mind bringing itself back to the moment. My mind's momentum had shifted so that it now wanted to stay present.

The Buddha said that the mind is the forerunner of all things. We create our worlds through what we practice. We choose to practice many of the skills we develop in our lives; others develop unconsciously. The qualities we cultivate can be external—skills such as playing music, engaging in athletics, reading, or writing. We can also develop internal qualities, such as love, joy, anger, jealousy, sadness, and generosity. Cultivating any pattern requires mindfulness, intention, and lots of practice.

Each stage of practice, from unconscious incompetence to unconscious competence, allows us to gather the wisdom and skill needed to fulfill our intentions. As arduous as practice can be in the early stages, there is no substitute for it, and the opportunities for learning throughout the process are infinite.

The stages of practice are fluid. Their boundaries are not sharp and defined. Often we find ourselves practicing within a particular stage without knowing how we got there. We sometimes move back and forth among the stages. In any discipline we endeavor to master, we will experience plateaus, which eventually give way to new vistas. Often these new vistas require that we move back into the earlier stages of practice in order to fully integrate the new skills required. At these times, the stages of practice become amorphous.

What are you are practicing now in your life? We become competent in whatever we practice, from the biggest, most elaborate skill to the subtlest internal states. Each stage of learning has value; we cannot skip any steps along the way. Effort begets effortlessness. Commit your attention to all aspects of your evolution; even the most seemingly insignificant details of the process can yield great insight. Wisdom grows as we commit our consciousness to each step. Let practice become your art.

Reflections

- Consider a discipline you've chosen to master in your life. Can you remember and identify the four stages of learning you went through as you developed your skills?

- Remember this model as you take up future practices, including the ones suggested in this book. Look back at this chapter as you begin to explore the eight limbs of yoga.

Right Effort: 4
Not Too Tight, Not Too Loose

THE FIRST DAYS of a meditation retreat are usually the time when my body complains the most. In some traditions, adjusting your body to lessen painful sensations is tantamount to cheating. Early on, I learned that in order to be a good yogi I had to sit perfectly still and simply experience the pain. Sitting unmoving for hours while enduring excruciating pain is heroic, I thought. The fact that I resisted squirming seemed even more virtuous when I knew that moving a fraction of an inch would likely alleviate the pain entirely.

So when, on the third day of a thirty-day retreat some years ago, my body felt as if it was on fire, I resolved to continue sitting no matter what. I sat for several hours with gritted teeth and stoic determination. This pain would not get the best of me, no matter how excruciating it became. It wasn't until nausea appeared in the third hour that I conceded and allowed myself to move a bit.

Sitting for almost three hours was my choice; the required sitting periods were actually only forty-five minutes. But I reasoned that surely if sitting for forty-five minutes is good, three hours must be better, and this would certainly prove me to be one of the more advanced yogis on the retreat. At that point, a tiny, unformed feeling of unease arose. Something seemed a bit off. What exactly was so heroic about sitting until one becomes nauseated?

Later in the retreat, we listened to a taped discourse in which Osho talked at length about the Herculean effort he had made in the early years of his practice. For many years he studied and practiced with such intensity that he eventually became so exhausted that he gave up. It was at that point, when he surrendered and stopped pushing himself, that what he had sought finally appeared to him.

The talk struck me like lightning. A wave of relief washed over me. In a single moment, I experienced all the years of conditioning wrought by living with my Depression-era father, a self-made man, for whom hard work—and not just hard work, but working harder than everyone else—was the centerpiece of creating a happy and worthwhile life. I remembered all the ways I had run myself to exhaustion in my daily life. A joyous truth washed through me: I don't have to work so hard!

I reported this experience to Pujari, who suggested that the rest of my retreat be dedicated to giving myself permission to rest. It was not hard work but ease that I needed to learn. I settled back, adjusted myself for comfort, and actually enjoyed the rest of the retreat. I realized that right effort can come in many guises.

In his book *The Heart of the Buddha's Teaching*, Thich Nhat Hanh tells a traditional Buddhist story about the teachings on effort. In the story the Buddha asks a musician monk, Sona, a musical question.

Thich Nhat Hanh writes: "The Buddha asked, 'What happens if the string of your instrument is too loose?'

'When you pluck it, there will be no sound,' Sona replied.

'What happens when the string is too taut?'

'It will break.'

'The practice of the Way is the same,' the Buddha said. 'Maintain your health. Be joyful. Do not force yourself to do things you cannot do.' "

In the same way, we can balance our own efforts in whatever we do. Whether the Way for you is meditation or yoga, playing a musical instrument, raising children, or going about your daily work, there exists a constant play between the sluggishness of sloth and the brittleness of over-effort. The Buddha spoke of right effort as one of the steps along the eightfold path.

After realizing my tendency to apply more effort than was necessary, I devoted the rest of my retreat to learning how to use effort in a skillful way. I found that my body operates in cycles that are fairly predictable. During certain periods of each day, there is a wealth of energy available. At other times, my energy is more flat. I found that when I respected my body's rhythms I could easily apply effort in more appropriate and effective ways than when I ignored my body's natural cycles.

For example, many people experience a drop in energy in the early afternoon. For this reason, many cultures build siesta time into their day. I found that during this time of lower energy I had several choices. I could continue applying massive effort, hoping that I could somehow push myself through the lethargy. This choice almost always produced feelings of frustration and even greater fatigue. I could also make lethargy the object of my meditation. Sometimes the energy of acceptance and observation caused tiredness to shift. Another choice was to awaken energy by taking a walk. At times when my efforts did not generate the energy to continue, I gave myself permission to take a nap, and to do so without the burden of guilt.

During times when energy was abundant, I challenged myself. I found that sometimes it was appropriate to sit for long periods. Often the energy I applied to meditation produced even more energy. The retreat became a laboratory for learning how to use effort skillfully.

The next challenge came when it was time to balance my responsibilities. It is a challenge that continues even now. In twenty-first-century American culture, having a full schedule is considered a sign of virtue, and taking time to relax, a sign of weakness or sloth. It is nice to feel that our lives are full and purposeful, but living in a state of constant activity, leaving no time to slow down and relax, does not promote balance. Balance is the ever-changing center point between action and rest. It is from this center point that we live most gracefully in the world.

I am as guilty as anyone of overloading my schedule with too many commitments. Not even a year after I'd begun dismantling my striving habit in meditation, I noticed that I was creating a great deal of stress from my inability to say no to worldly commitments. Even though I was learning to balance my effort in meditation, the skill had not yet integrated into my life. Well-practiced habits do not easily fade away. As Pujari once told me, "Even after you've stopped pedaling a bicycle, it still coasts along for a while." I saw each new commitment as an opportunity, and many of them were. But opportunities quickly become burdens when there are too many of them. For about six months, I literally ran from my house to my car and from my car to my appointments.

I had also developed a habit of doing several things at once—mostly talking on the phone while washing dishes, sweeping the floor, or weeding the garden. Sometimes I even talked on the phone while checking and writing e-mail, guaranteeing inattentiveness in both communications. I was simply going through the motions, which made my work ultimately unsatisfying. The fact that my work no longer felt enjoyable generated more stress. As full as my life was, it felt quite empty.

One day I was driving to a meeting with a potential employer. Grumpy from exhaustion, I was grousing to myself about the schedule I'd set up. Suddenly a woman ran a red light and broadsided my car in the middle of a busy intersection. My car spun around, and my head smashed into the side window. I sustained a concussion, whiplash, and a laceration that required seven stitches.

For six months following the accident, I could not lower my head below my heart without feeling as if it might explode—quite a limiting handicap for someone who practices and teaches asana. I had no idea whether I'd ever again be able to practice basic poses such as Adho Mukha Svanasana (Downward-Facing Dog Pose), let alone my very favorite pose, Salamba Sarvangasana (Shoulderstand).

At the time, I also had a part-time job as editor of publications for a private school. For the first four weeks after my injury, I could not read. I could comprehend individual words, but my mind could not retain them long enough to string them together into a sentence. At the time, I wondered whether I would ever read again. And I was profoundly exhausted. Most days I slept at least twelve hours. I had to drop almost everything. My fatigue was so deep and my short-term memory so fragmented that I could not keep track of my complicated life. The only responsibility I retained during the first few weeks was to teach my asana classes.

I was surprised to see that my life unfolded quite smoothly, even when I had—albeit unintentionally—completely relinquished most of my responsibilities. The myriad little details of life that had kept me racing were not as earth-shatteringly important as I'd thought. At that point, I resolved that I would never again overload my schedule so that I had to sprint from one thing to the next.

Sometimes even now I fall back into overscheduling myself. The difference now is that I make sure the busyness is finite. After a particularly frenzied week or two, I always give myself a do-nothing day. I take short breaks during even the busiest days. Incorporating even small amounts of slow, mindful movements into the day can align us more closely with our balance point. Shifting out of work mode, even for short periods, might even increase our ability to accomplish what we need to do. When I take time each day to drop my schedule and do something completely unrelated to work or to do nothing at all, I come back to my responsibilities with more clarity and equanimity.

On the more tightly scheduled days, I might simply take a leisurely walk around the block, practice one or two yoga asanas, wash the dishes with extra care, weed a small section of my garden, play with my cats, prepare a meal, or enjoy a cup of tea. I make a point to perform these actions more slowly than my usual pace and with complete presence. This calms me and gives rise to a quiet happiness. When my mind settles in this way, fulfilling my commitments becomes a pleasure.

What are the signals that you are working too hard? Resentment, tightness, anger, and frustration may be signs that you need to back off your efforts. You may also notice that your breathing is shallow, labored, or erratic. When these conditions are present, you might consider stopping, taking a few deep breaths, and calming your approach. Or maybe lay down your project and shift your attention to something else for a while.

On the other hand, when effort is lacking, you can feel sluggish, unfocused, unable to finish what you have set out to do. At these times, asserting some effort can sometimes arouse energy. This can be challenging when it seems there is no reserve from which to draw energy. Taking a brisk walk often can generate focus and vitality. A few minutes of mindful asana practice or deep breathing can yield the energy you need.

Asana practice is the perfect laboratory to explore the quality of your effort. In each asana, the quality of effort needed will vary. It will also vary from day to day. In order to practice in a balanced way, you must shift your intention from accomplishing the pose to finding and exploring your edge. When your intention in asana practice is to place your head on your knee in a forward bend or to accomplish a more intense backbend, your effort almost always will be too much. On a physiological level, you will likely create more tension in the body rather than less.

Conversely, when you find your mind always making excuses not to try something new or challenging, your efforts likely are unbalanced in the direction of lethargy. You may need to arouse energy by resolving to move gently and mindfully beyond what you believe your boundaries to be. When you practice with balance in mind, it doesn't matter how your asana looks. A person who is inflexible will receive the same benefit as one who is very flexible.

How can you begin to practice with balance as the intention? You can practice balance by finding the edge where you feel challenged but where there is still space in the body–mind to relax. There is energy to go deeper, along with the understanding that going deeper means relaxing into the current challenge.

The breath is the most effective gauge for balancing effort with ease in asana practice. When the breathing becomes shallow, erratic, or nonexistent, you are likely doing too much. At these times, you are sending signals through the nervous system that the body is in danger. The nervous system responds by tightening the muscles further. Practice so that the breath is calm, deep, and in harmony with the outer manifestation of the asana. Then the body can relax.

Finding balance is a moment-by-moment process. With each breath, your experience of the asana changes. When you allow the mind to listen to your body, rather than letting it dictate what you should do or feel, effort begins to rectify itself naturally.

Exploring the quality of your effort in asana practice is instructive and supportive of how you approach the challenges of your life. What you discover on the mat is indicative of patterns you practice in life. And what you practice on the mat will affect how you respond to challenges in your life. No matter what you are doing, you can always check in with your breath, noting whether there is ease or unease there.

The chapters that follow give exercises for exploring the concepts I've presented so far. Some of these exercises may resonate for you; others may not. Practice the ones that seem right for you, without hurrying to practice all of them. A year or two from now, you may find yourself drawn to some that you don't connect with now. Practice only one or two at a time, so you can give each your complete attention.

At its essence, the practice of right effort means learning to act in harmony with the truth. It is the vehicle through which you can accomplish your goals in a way that respects the energy you have available at any given moment. When your actions are in harmony with what is true for you, you feel joy and ease in everything you do.

Reflections

- Take time after each asana to notice what you feel. What is the quality of your breath? Do you feel agitated or calm? What is the quality of your final relaxation at the end of practice? When you have practiced with right effort, your practice feels complete; you feel both relaxed and energized. When effort is out of balance, you often feel residual agitation or fatigue.

- If you tend to overschedule, make a list of your commitments. Prioritize them in order of importance. Are there any responsibilities you can let go, at least for a day or two? Communicate with others about your intentions, if necessary. What feelings arise at the thought of relinquishing just one of your duties for a day or two? Any time you feel overwhelmed, revisit this practice.

- Take time in the middle of your day to put down your work and do something completely different, even for five or ten minutes. Take a walk; have a cup of tea. Practice a slow, relaxing asana, or take long, deep breaths. Do this for a month. At the end of the month, note any shifts in your attitudes toward your work and toward your few minutes of downtime.

Part iii

Walking Your Path

The Eight Limbs of Yoga: 5
The Yoga of Living

A STORY FROM the time of the Buddha tells of a hapless frog who came upon a dharma talk being given by the master himself. While hearing the voice of the Buddha, which was said to be sweet and resonant as well as wise and compassionate, the unfortunate frog was inadvertently smashed and killed by the walking staff of a human listener. Because the frog was hearing the dharma delivered by the Buddha at the powerful moment of his transition from life to death, he was instantly enlightened and catapulted to the *deva* realm, one of the heavenly realms of existence.

Buddhist lore is rich with tales of monks who reached full enlightenment within weeks of beginning practice while in the presence of the Buddha. The monk Ananda awakened to the infinite as he lay down to sleep one night. Modern-day stories of instant awakening exist as well. In her book *Collision with the Infinite*, the late Suzanne Segal chronicles her story of a sudden shift into what she termed "the vastness" while stepping onto a bus. Eckhart Tolle, former Cambridge University research scholar and best-selling author of *The Power of Now*, leapt into the timeless one night while lying in bed.

Stories of instant enlightenment are inspiring. While it is true that freedom is possible for all of us at any moment, most of us awaken gradually. In the same way that water eventually fills a bucket one drop at a time, each small step along our path contributes to our awakening. Those who are catapulted to freedom need no roadmap. For the rest of us, wise beings throughout history have provided many and varied step-by-step instructions for treading the path of awakening. The Buddha outlined what he eightfold path. The path includes right view, right thinking, right ᴤight action, right livelihood, right effort, right mindfulness, and ᴤcentration. Understanding and practicing the principles of the eightᴤ.ᴤd path is a lifelong learning process, each step awakening us gradually to the truth of who we are. This path encompasses all aspects of our lives. Indeed, there is no area of living that is outside the spiritual.

In the second and third chapters of the Yoga Sutras, Patanjali outlines an eight-limbed path to awakening. While the organization of the eightfold path and eight limbs of yoga are quite different, many of the same principles abide within each system. Patanjali's explanation of the eight-limbed path to *samadhi* begins in the second *pada* (chapter) of the Yoga Sutras, the chapter titled "Sadhana Pada" in Sanskrit, or "Treading the Path."

I first learned of the eight limbs of yoga in 1989, while studying for my teaching certification in the Iyengar system of yoga. At the time, I gave these principles the same kind of cursory attention I had given my studies in college—the minimum needed to pass the exam. I was quite resistant to learning yoga philosophy because I believed it to be a religion, and I did not want to be confined by it. Nor did I want to force a philosophy onto my students, one that might interfere with their personal beliefs.

Because most of my teaching had been in Salt Lake City, I was especially sensitive to the problems inherent in presenting anything remotely spiritual to a population whose culture is heavily influenced by a particular religion. Many of my students were raised in the Church of Jesus Christ of Latter Day Saints (LDS). I did not want to present anything that might be perceived as challenging to or disrespectful of beliefs they held dear. I felt that many of my non-LDS students, especially those who had grown up in an LDS-dominated culture, might also be alienated by what could be perceived as an attempt to influence their beliefs. Presenting yoga as a nonsectarian physical discipline severed from its spiritual context seemed safer for my students and for myself.

Meanwhile I continued to learn Buddhist principles, all of which pointed to experiences all humans share. When I began to look more closely at the Yoga Sutras, I realized that they too are based in universal understanding that is compatible with all belief systems. The eight limbs of yoga, as presented by Patanjali in the Yoga Sutras, are simply a set of guidelines that can be interpreted within the context of any spiritual system or on their own, unconfined by any beliefs. The limbs are designed to guide each person in his or her own way. There are as many ways to manifest the eight-limbed system of yoga as there are people.

In the introduction to his book *The Yoga Sutras of Patanjali*, Alistair Shearer writes: "Whether we choose to practice yoga, and interpret its benefits, within the framework of a conventional set of religious beliefs is up to us. Some people do, some don't. Yoga itself is neutral. It is a catalyst that allows us to grow in whichever direction is natural and life-supporting. Its methods work on the physical seat of consciousness, the nervous system, and, as far as yoga is concerned, a Hindu nervous system is no different from an Islamic or agnostic one. Each obeys the same laws that govern the operations of mind and body. Whoever practices yoga will be enlivened in his or her own way."

Yoga means "union." In the West, this is interpreted as the union of mind and body. While that interpretation is correct, the unification that takes place as we practice the eight-limbed path can also be seen as an integration of all the aspects of our lives. Asana practice by itself can reap marvelous benefits. Practiced in the context of the eight limbs, yoga becomes a guide for living.

The limbs relate to each other in the same way as the limbs on our bodies do. Rather than being hierarchical, the limbs extend out from and feed into a central, whole being: ourselves. Rather than being separate concepts, the limbs connect to one another. The practice of one limb influences and strengthens all the others.

The eight limbs address all aspects of practice, most important that practice that takes place in our daily lives. Every aspect of the system is designed to bring us closer to the heart of yoga, the settling of the mind into stillness. Far from being esoteric principles that are available only to a few special, spiritual people, the eight-limbed path can be applied to anyone's life. Practicing the eight limbs of yoga strengthens and enhances our understanding of our practice and our lives.

Patanjali's eight limbs are:

1. Yama: ethical principles
   Ahimsa: nonharming

Satya: truth

Asteya: nonstealing

Brahmacharya: conservation of energy, wise use of sexuality

Aparigraha: nongreed, generosity

2. Niyama: personal practices

Saucha: cleanliness, purity

Santosha: contentment

Tapas: discipline, enthusiasm, simplicity

Svadhyaya: study of the self, study of spiritual texts

Ishvarapranidhana: surrender to grace

3. Asana: the practice of physical postures

4. Pranayama: expansion of the life force through refinement of the breath

5. Pratyahara: refinement of the senses

6. Dharana: concentration

7. Dhyana: meditation

8. Samadhi: the completely settled mind

The eight-limbed path is a path of action. Before embarking on your journey, it is helpful to set an intention. The intention might be to focus on one limb each month or one limb each year. You might decide to study the limbs formally within the context of all the sutras. You might enjoy practicing the yamas in the context of your asana practice, or practicing the niyamas as a meditation. Choose and commit to an intention that fits your life in an honest and practical way.

The eight-limbed path is a lifelong practice. As you travel along the path, your understanding of the limbs will become increasingly refined. Sometimes it will be necessary to revise interpretations that once felt appropriate in order for new insight to arise. Because the eight limbs apply to all aspects of our lives, they are infinitely enriching on all levels. Reflecting on how each limb applies to your own life helps solidify understanding.

The chapters that follow reflect my personal understanding of the limbs at this point in my journey. In my readings of the Yoga Sutras and the eight limbs, I have found that there are many ways of understanding these concepts. Each author presents different ideas and interpretations, which makes great fodder for your own exploration. Please consider my words in the context of your own life experience. If a concept I present does not fit for you, I encourage you to read other books that address the eight limbs.

In these chapters, explanations of each limb are accompanied by suggestions for how to integrate the teachings into your life. Each of the suggested practices is meant to be savored, perhaps practiced over a long period of time. Do not try to practice everything at once. It may feel appropriate to work with a practice for a while, let it go, and then return to it somewhere down the road.

Most important, use your experience as your guide to uncover your own truth. No single person's life experience can ever match another's. Walking the eight-limbed path leads us into the heart of our own unique truth. Clarify your intent, and let your journey begin.

The First Limb
Yama: Living in Harmony with All Beings

6

ULTIMATELY ALL BEINGS share the same life. We live together on this fertile planet sustaining ourselves with its gifts—earth, water, air, and sunshine. All animals, including humans, nourish their bodies with the fruits, vegetables, and grains rooted in the earth. The decay of flora and fauna replenishes the soil, which then sprouts new life. What we exhale, the trees around us inhale; what the trees exhale, we inhale. The earth's resources sustain our lives, and we share in the responsibility to care for those resources for the benefit of all.

When we care for our planet and its inhabitants, we are also caring for ourselves. This is because all who share this earth are interconnected. Often we can see clearly and immediately how the actions we choose in the world affect our lives. But what we do also yields effects that are far-reaching and unfathomable. A concept called the butterfly effect illustrates the power of our actions. According to this idea, when a butterfly flutters its wings, it creates an air current. This air current resounds not only throughout the butterfly's immediate environment but it cascades out, gathering momentum as it interacts with the atmosphere. Eventually it becomes strong enough to alter weather patterns on the far side of the world.

In the same way, our daily choices create effects in the world that we may never know. This may be the most important reason for embarking on a path of awakening. When we are conscious of our motivations, we can choose wisely. When we choose wisely, our lives and the lives of those around us are more harmonious. We cannot know how many lives we nourish by living consciously.

In 1993 the National Demonstration Project to Reduce Violent Crime and Improve Governmental Effectiveness conducted an experiment in Washington, D.C. The study brought four thousand students of the Transcendental Meditation and TM-Sidhi programs to the capital city for two months to help reduce stress through group meditations. At the end of the period, the study found a significant reduction in violent crimes correlated with the size of the study group, which varied from week to week. In the final week, when the number of participants peaked, the study recorded its highest percentage decrease in violent crime at 23.3 percent.

In the beginning and in the end, the fruits of our practice are manifest most significantly in how we live. The amazing physical feats we perform on the yoga mat mean little if we are not carrying consciousness into our daily work and relationships. This is why precepts for ethical behavior are the cornerstone of every spiritual system. The first limb of yoga, as outlined by Patanjali, is *yama*, five guidelines for living harmoniously in the world, which include nonharming; truth; nonstealing; wise use of energy, including sexual energy; and nongreed, or generosity. The mind is not likely to settle into stillness if our relationships are in disharmony.

Traditionally yoga is introduced by study, contemplation, and practice of the yamas and niyamas before or at least in concert with the beginning of asana practice. In an interview about teaching yoga to children, Swati and Rajiv Chanchani discussed the importance of building a foundation for practice based in the yamas and niyamas. "Yoga is more than yogasanas," said Swati. "So part of yoga is the upbringing. [Children] are taught the food, the lifestyle . . . More important than the yogasanas are the yamas and niyamas, and the whole yogic lifestyle and worldview."

The Buddha outlined five precepts, almost identical to the yamas of Patanjali, which he taught as a basis for practice. About these precepts Jack Kornfield writes, "The positive power of virtue is enormous. When we don't live by these precepts, it is said we live like wild beasts; without them, all other spiritual practice is a sham. Imagine trying to sit down and meditate after lying and stealing. Then imagine what a different world this would be if everyone kept even one precept—not to kill, or not to lie, or not to steal. We would truly create a new world order."

We can see how the limbs of yoga practice relate to each other in our practice of the yamas. When we endeavor to behave ethically in the world, there is less agitation present in the mind. Just as we can see to the bottom of a lake when its water is still, when we quiet the mind we see the situations that arise in our lives with greater clarity and can make wiser choices. Our worldly relationships are a reflection of our practice. When we cultivate our minds through practice, our lives become more peaceful; as our lives become more peaceful, our minds settle.

As with all the eight limbs, practicing the yamas is a lifelong process of refinement. After several years of asana practice, you might notice that your body has changed and is able to relax more deeply into certain postures that may have previously seemed impossible. In the same way, we continually refine our understanding of the yamas as we act within their framework. It is easy to look back from our present level of understanding and see how we might have behaved differently in the past, if only we knew then what we know now. This is a natural part of our evolution; it tells us that we are indeed evolving.

The yamas are guidelines, a framework from which we can begin a process of inquiry. They are not commandments, nor are they intended to be followed mechanically. Practicing the yamas simply because they are written in the sutras does not lead us to greater wisdom. Understanding of the yamas comes from considering them in the context of each situation that arises in our lives and being mindful of the consequences of our actions.

As in all other practices, we will sometimes stumble or fall. Conscious reflection helps us to see where we might have altered our behavior. The yamas are like any other skill we want to develop: We must practice. Over time, with conscious practice, our understanding of the yamas becomes more refined.

When people embark upon a formal Buddhist practice, they begin by committing to follow the five ethical precepts outlined by the Buddha. In the same way, as we commit to practice yoga we can set the intention to let the yamas guide our life choices. Jack Kornfield describes the evolutionary process of practicing the precepts. "At first, precepts are a practice. Then they become a necessity, and finally they become a joy. When our heart is awakened, they spontaneously illuminate our way in the world. This is called Shining Virtue. The light around someone who speaks truth, who consistently acts with compassion for all, even in great difficulty, is visible to all around them."

Sutra I.1, as translated by Alistair Shearer, says: "And now the teaching on yoga begins." At first glance I discounted this sutra as a throwaway verse. In revisiting it later in my sutra study, I saw this verse as the setting of intention. Intention is the impulse that precedes all action and colors everything we undertake. When we see our intentions clearly, we can more easily determine whether actions we are considering will bring happiness or harm.

For example: I feel an impulse to share. My motivation might be political—I'd like to ingratiate myself with someone because she has something to offer me. Another motivation might simply be the impulse to give, free of any expectation. While the act of giving is virtually the same in both scenarios, differing motivations color the results. Knowing our intentions can help us understand the possible fruits of our actions. As we grow in mindfulness, we see our intentions more clearly and can make choices accordingly.

The only moral dictum I ever heard my parents repeat (and they did so frequently) was the golden rule: "Do unto others as you would have them do unto you." The yamas can be seen as specific guidelines that teach us how to practice this universal precept. When we are faced with a moral question in our lives, it can be helpful to consider the possible viewpoints of all beings involved. The next time you have a difficult decision to make that will affect someone else, put yourself in the other person's place. When you reverse your perspective, note what you feel. What emotions arise? Can you accomplish what you want in a way that is sensitive to the needs of everyone? Changing your viewpoint can help you clarify a skillful course of action.

We are not alone in this world, and everything we do has an impact. Being aware of the yamas and solidifying our intention to practice from their foundation allows us to live wisely and compassionately. The fruit borne through actions rooted in the yamas is sweet, nourishing the earth and all its inhabitants.

Reflections

- Choose one yama to practice for a period of time—a week, a month, or a year. At the end of that time, decide whether you'd like to continue with the same principle or if its momentum is strong enough that you'd like to add another. As always, be patient. The yamas are lifelong practices. Watch how they evolve. You may even want to write down your observations about your practice. Review your observations periodically, and note what you've learned.

Ahimsa: 7
Dynamic Peacefulness

MAHATMA GANDHI said that nonviolence is the greatest force at the disposal of mankind. Jesus encouraged his followers to love their enemies. The Buddha taught that hatred never ceases by hatred but ceases only through love, according to the ancient law.

The philosophies of virtually every spiritual system in this world share one common ground: the intention to not cause harm. The foundation of nonharming is active cultivation of the love that illuminates all aspects of our lives and protects us from the tendency to act from anger or ill will. The ability to love without condition—our friends, colleagues, and families, as well as those who would harm us—is our greatest challenge, our greatest power, our greatest joy.

Ahimsa, or nonviolence, is the first of the yamas, and the foundation upon which all of yogic life is balanced. All the other yamas grow from ahimsa. Each of the yamas carries within it the intention of creating respectful and loving relationships with our fellow beings. Ahimsa honors all life: great and small, human and nonhuman, animal and plant, earth, sky, and water. This precept asks us to consider the consequences of our actions to ourselves and to the world around us.

Alistair Shearer describes ahimsa as "a dynamic peacefulness that is prepared to meet all situations with a loving openness." The phrase "dynamic peacefulness" suggests an ever-shifting state of quiet balance, a constantly changing, evolving equanimity that allows us to meet each situation in our lives individually, rather than mechanically or habitually. It also puts forward the idea that peacefulness is not necessarily a static or passive state. Practicing ahimsa requires that we be aware of and engaged with the world around us. Sometimes ahimsa moves us to take action to alleviate the suffering in our world.

Ahimsa is a quality that arises from within, a state that we come from. It is a characteristic that, though intrinsic to all of us, can be developed through intention and practice. Mindful awareness is a key faculty here, as it allows us to see our motivations with clarity and to act from our highest potential. As we orient ourselves to living peacefully, we become peace. Like all aspects of yoga, ahimsa is a quality that we cultivate and refine throughout our lives.

The practice of ahimsa begins with our relationship to ourselves. All of our other relationships reflect how we feel about ourselves. Those qualities we judge most harshly in ourselves are also the ones we find least tolerable in others. It is quite helpful, although not always pleasant, to note what judgments we hold about ourselves. Note your self-talk, both positive and negative. When you think about yourself, do you picture a whole, multifaceted person, or do you see only the qualities you like, or those that you don't?

I first observed my own deeply ingrained judging habit on a ten-day vipassana meditation retreat in 1988. I saw how nothing in my experience escaped my constant evaluation. I judged each breath, each sitting meditation, each bite of food, each step I took, as being good or bad. I even judged my judgments, and judged myself for judging. Of course I judged the other retreat participants as well. One person seemed sad, one person seemed arrogant, another was too noisy, another seemed just a little too good to be true.

The pervasiveness of my judging habit astounded me. The suffering that came from constant judgment was undeniable. The feeling that accompanied rampant judging was one of tightness and irritation. Judgment obscured and reduced everything in my experience. In seeing the pattern so clearly, I was able to begin the arduous process of dismantling it. In chipping away at my judging habit, my vision of the world around me has become larger and more colorful, not the cramped, black-and-white universe I inhabited when everything had to be reduced to "good" or "bad."

What judgments do you carry about yourself and others? How do they affect your ability to perceive your experience clearly?

We are all a constellation of many qualities—some that we like and others that we do not. It is essential for us to see ourselves in a holistic way and to recognize the many qualities that we share with others. We also can recognize our uniqueness and learn from our diversity. It is the understanding of our profound interrelatedness that inspires us to practice the yamas. When we see our interconnectedness clearly, it becomes more difficult to behave disrespectfully toward our world. It becomes impossible to litter the ground or deface a tree or kill an animal for sport.

Life offers us many opportunities to test our commitment to ahimsa. For several years I have taught asana classes on guided river rafting trips. Biting insects are an integral part of the river environment. In the spring the no-see-ums—gnatlike insects that swarm around your face—can be almost unbearable. One season when the no-see-ums were particularly populous I came home with more than forty bites on my face and neck alone. One woman on the trip suffered a severe anaphylactic reaction to the bites. No amount of insect repellent deterred them.

It was very tempting to swat them as they swarmed around my face and lit in my dinner. But finally I chose to let them be. First, I realized the absolute futility of swatting them. One or two dead no-see-ums—or one or two hundred—would not have made any difference in the number of bites I sustained. Then I realized that I was visiting their environment, and it is their nature to seek sustenance. We humans are an easily accessible source of nourishment. Seeking a peaceful solution, I returned home and bought a mosquito net that has served nicely on subsequent river trips.

I once heard the story of a blind monk who lived in the time of the Buddha. While practicing his walking meditation, he would inadvertently step on ants, killing them. Seeing the blind monk causing the ants harm, a group of monks became upset and went to the Buddha. They asked him how this monk could be allowed to practice when he was breaking the first precept of nonharming. The Buddha pointed out the difference between a person who deliberately steps on ants and a blind monk who simply cannot see them. The distinction lay in the intention.

The diet we choose can express our intention not to harm. My body happens to thrive on a plant-based diet. As a child eating the typical American four-food-group diet, I suffered from chronic abdominal pain and stomach upset. My body was simply unable to digest meat efficiently. When I stopped eating meat in 1978, I was amazed at the difference. Not only did my digestive problems clear up completely, but my energy rose to levels I'd never felt before. I feel fortunate that the diet that best suits my body allows me to practice ahimsa in a way that is meaningful to me, given my love for animals.

Animals are our fellow travelers on this planet. Despite the habits of our culture, they do not exist solely for our exploitation. Their existence has intrinsic worth. In the interest of expediency and profit, Western culture has embraced the practice of factory farming, which causes animals to spend their lives in conditions of overcrowding and malnutrition. Mahatma Gandhi said that a nation and its moral progress can be judged by the way it treats its animals. The existence of factory farming is a reminder that as a culture we have a lot to learn.

There are, however, people living in parts of the world where there is no other choice but to eat meat much of the time. Those who live in climates where ice and snow cover the ground most of the year maintain their health by consuming the flesh and fat of animals they catch. Years ago I saw a film called *Atanarjuat: The Fast Runner*. The film recounts a traditional Inuit legend and portrays the relentlessly icy environment of northern Alaska. As I watched the film, which shows the Inuit people catching and skinning animals for food, I reflected on the fact that had they not eaten meat the people would have starved. There were no other options. Tibet's high-altitude environment is also such a place. For this reason, Tibetan Buddhism does not promote strict vegetarianism. Because their choices are limited, Tibetans would likely suffer malnutrition or starvation if they did not eat meat.

There are also people in more hospitable climates whose bodies operate better when they ingest animal protein. Many of these people have food sensitivities that leave them with very few other options for obtaining protein. It can be argued that denying our bodies nutrients they need also causes harm. When we attempt to force strict vegetarianism on ourselves or others, are we not practicing a form of violence?

If you are a person whose body needs animal protein but you would rather not eat meat, dairy products and eggs might be the answer. If your body simply needs the flesh of animals to sustain it, can you find a meat source that does not engage in cruel or unhealthy practices? If not, perhaps you might take a moment before eating to honor the animal that has shared its life with you. Reflecting on where your nourishment comes from can reconnect you with the truth of your interrelatedness with all living beings.

The sutra that describes ahimsa (II.35) says (in Shearer's translation), "When we are firmly established in nonviolence, all beings around us cease to feel hostility." Because of our intrinsic interconnectedness with other beings, whatever we have integrated in our lives naturally radiates out and touches those around us. When ahimsa becomes integrated into our own being, we radiate the light of kindness and compassion. Others can feel safe and relaxed in our presence, without the fear that underlies harmful actions.

Cultivating ahimsa doesn't mean that we don't sometimes feel anger, jealousy, or aversion. But in practicing ahimsa we learn to respond to those emotions without cultivating even more judgment and aversion. Violence always begets more violence. When we respond to our negative emotions with more negativity, we continue the cycle of harming; we reinforce the habit. Part of the practice is to meet our own challenges with acceptance. We accept that difficult emotions are present in a way that neither indulges nor suppresses them.

Acceptance of all parts of ourselves is the key to cultivating compassion for all beings. We must know and accept ourselves completely before we can accept others fully. Mindfulness practice is invaluable here. As we look deeply at what is present in our experience, we develop the spaciousness of mind to accept what we see.

There are many different ways to bring the practice of ahimsa into our lives. Notice if you reflexively kill insects you find living in your home. Instead of immediately squashing the next bug you find, you might ask yourself, Is the intruder really causing harm where it is? If so, is there a way I can humanely trap it and escort it outdoors?

Our buying choices can be an expression of ahimsa. Perhaps you live in a place where you readily can buy products that do not cause harm—fair-trade coffee, cruelty-free cosmetics, clothing not assembled in sweat shops, items sold by companies that treat their employees fairly, organic products that do not harm the environment.

Depending on where you live and what resources you have to spend, you may not be able to do this. If that is the case, it's best not to cause further harm by judging yourself. Do whatever you can in other areas of your life. Being kind to your family and friends is a wonderful way to practice ahimsa—in thoughts, words, and actions.

The most important thing is to be aware of your intentions and actions. At first that can seem like a lot of work, but as with everything you practice, after a while conscious choice becomes natural. It becomes a habit. As you look at your life, in what areas could you refine your actions to do less harm?

Sometimes ahimsa calls us to activism. Is there a cause you'd like to help out? Often it is anger or frustration that motivates us to act. Ahimsa asks us to do the painstaking work of uncovering the love that invariably lies beneath the surface of anger and frustration, so we can act from a ground of good will.

Because all the yamas are rooted in ahimsa, discussions of the other precepts might help you define areas in your life where you have cultivated wise choices and others that have yet to be explored. As you read about the yamas, remember that you have come to where you are today by walking a path that is unique to you. Use the discussions that follow to honor your own practice and to integrate practice of the yamas in a way that fits the landscape of your own journey.

Ahimsa in Your Asana Practice

Asana practice is the perfect forum for cultivating ahimsa. The mindfulness that accompanies asana practice allows us to see when and how we judge ourselves on the basis of what our bodies can or cannot do. These judgments are either deflating or inflating at best and injurious at worst. Sometimes these judgments simply make us feel negative about ourselves. Other times they motivate us to force our bodies into positions that harm them.

Watch the thoughts that arise in your practice, especially when you feel you are not doing your "best" pose. Asana practice is not about performance. Can you practice from a ground of dynamic peacefulness? Can you relinquish the goal of physical accomplishment for the intention of cultivating peace?

Reflections

■ Take time each day to reflect on the kind or generous acts you've done in that day. Consider the many wonderful gifts you've been given by your friends, family, and teachers. Practice this daily for a month or longer. Notice if and how this practice influences your feelings about yourself and others.

■ Refine your buying choices, such as buying organic foods or cruelty-free products.

■ In 1993, after emerging from an emotionally difficult time, I struggled a lot with anger and ill will. I talked to Pujari, who gave me an "emotional map" to follow. It was so helpful that I share it with you.

Navigating the map requires only that you be fully present for whatever emotion is arising. As you remain aware of the emotions you encounter in each layer and allow them to inhabit you for as long as they are present, they eventually dissolve to reveal the layer that exists underneath. Again, inhabit these emotions as they arise. Stay with each layer of emotion as long as it is present and again, when it dissolves, identify and be with what is next revealed.

Begin by choosing a comfortable position. You may want to lie down or sit in a chair or on a meditation cushion. You can also practice this while walking. Choose a position that best suits your present situation. For example, if you feel agitated, you may want to practice slow walking to help steady your energy. Sitting with your back supported might be appropriate if you feel that walking creates greater agitation. The best position for this process is the one that feels kindest to your body.

The surface layer is often anger, blame, or resentment. Become aware of anger and all its attendant sensations, especially those that reside in the physical body. Stay with these emotions as long as they remain. When you penetrate the outer layer of anger, you may unearth hurt, sadness, and disappointment. Explore these feelings by entering them completely, noticing where they reside in the body and how they differ from the sensation of anger. Often underneath the hurt is fear and insecurity. As you move through fear and insecurity, you might find remorse and regret. Here you can take responsibility for your part in the difficulty. Once you have considered how you contributed to the situation, identify and set your intentions and wishes. When you reach the deepest level, you will find love, appreciation, understanding, and forgiveness. It is here where healing and transformation lie.

Use this map when you feel overwhelmed by emotion. You may need to visit the map more than once. Be patient. Notice the emotions that arise and allow the map to unfold in its own time. Investigating powerful emotions can be an interesting practice. When you feel angry at someone, let go of the repetitive thoughts that continue to feed the anger. Instead, become present with the sensation of anger, in particular how and where you feel it in your body. Notice if you are judging yourself for feeling angry. Begin to let go of the judgment.

It is important to allow each emotion to arise and dissolve in its own time. Avoid trying to hurry the process. Think of it as a journey of discovery; each step is as important as the next. Even a few minutes of practice are helpful. If you can devote twenty minutes or more to this practice, you are likely to observe great shifts in your emotional landscape.

Satya: 8
Impeccable Truthfulness

S ILENT VIPASSANA MEDITATION retreats are not completely silent. Every few days those attending are given an opportunity to talk one-on-one with their teacher for fifteen minutes. The interview, as it's called, is a time when one can ask questions, share experiences, or simply check in.

Early in my practice, I often skipped the interviews, telling myself that talking was too disruptive to my practice. But it was not the talking itself that was problematic. For hours before the interview, my meditation practice would be riddled with anxiety. What would I ask? Are my questions silly? What meditative experiences were appropriate to share? What could I talk about that would show that I was making progress? What could I say that would reflect me in a positive light? I spent hours mentally rehearsing the interview. More often than not, I opted to skip the interview altogether. This freed me from a great deal of anxiety and allowed me to concentrate on my practice.

In 1992 and 1993, I went through a very difficult time. For many months, I was trapped in a rotating and quite hellish kaleidoscope of insecurities, neuroses, and all the unhealthy patterns I had cultivated throughout my life. During this period I spoke with Pujari frequently and spent several weekends with him and Abhilasha in solo retreat at their cabin. I was feeling so raw, so desperate, that I did not have the luxury of planning my talks with Pujari in order to choose the most palatable details to share. Because I had no energy for artful communication, I became painfully honest in my interactions with all my friends and family. If I had edited out the unpleasant, there would have been no conversation.

The next time I attended a vipassana retreat, in 1994, I found to my surprise that I no longer felt intimidated by the interviews. The previous year had shown me that no matter what I shared, Pujari would respond with complete, nonjudgmental acceptance. I also found that honesty had not lost me any friends. I realized that no question was silly, no experience would be judged. I no longer felt a need to rehearse my interviews. Instead, I told the truth. I was surprised at how constructive the interviews became when I spoke freely and honestly. I was equally amazed at how simple it was to tell the truth, compared with all the agonizing machinations I went through trying to create and uphold an admirable image.

Of course, my pattern of rehearsing conversations was not confined to meditation retreats. Rehearsing possible future interactions was a well-developed habit. Detailed planning allowed me to feel confident that the image I projected was aligned with how I wanted to be seen. Rehearsing conversations—communications that more often than not never took place outside my own head—consumed an enormous amount of my mental energy. As I began to see the pattern clearly, I realized how much of my vitality was being dispersed by the desire to paint an image of myself that I felt would be favorable to others. Upholding an untrue image was exhausting and completely unnecessary. When I began to experience the simplicity of being honestly who I am without trying to project an image, I felt free. My life became less cluttered.

One of the great gifts of mindfulness practice is the opportunity to see clearly, like it or not, what patterns we habitually nurture in our lives. In the often chaotic process of living, it is easy to cruise along on automatic, mindlessly filtering our thought, speech, and action through well-established habits of behavior. When we become quiet for long enough, our habitual behaviors come to the fore, where we can watch them cycling endlessly, like familiar old tape loops set to play over and over.

This is one of the great challenges of meditation. These patterns can be supremely annoying. It's much easier to keep busy and allow the patterns to run without having to acknowledge their existence. The problem is, if we are not aware of them, these patterns of thought, behavior, and belief form an overlay through which we filter all our experience. The filters make it impossible to see the truth of what is present. Our vision of reality is colored and distorted until we identify those patterns that consistently obscure our sight.

When you understand that these habits no longer serve you, you can begin to dismantle them. First, you must acknowledge and accept the pattern. Then you can exercise your greatest power—the power to choose to feed the habit or not.

This is where *satya*, the second yama, begins. Satya is impeccable truthfulness in thoughts, words, and deeds. Like ahimsa, the practice of satya originates with our relationship to ourselves, in knowing ourselves completely. If we do not know who we are, how can we begin to form relationships based in truth? If we are not aware of the beliefs and thought patterns that color our experience, how can we listen to someone without overlaying our biases? How can we make wise and compassionate choices if we are not aware of our honest intentions?

Our thoughts, which are often projections or fantasies, often motivate our actions. The practice of satya begins with the careful observation of our thoughts and psychological patterns. When we can identify the beliefs and patterns through which we filter our experience, we can consider their influence—and unhook ourselves from it—as we make choices. As with all practices in the yogic life, satya is an evolving effort, one that sustains and supports all the other facets of our lives.

As we observe our thoughts and patterns carefully, we become increasingly adept at knowing the difference between projection and truth. Then we can choose to act from our core integrity and abandon actions that spring from projection. As with all yogic practices, our awareness, and therefore our ability to act with integrity, becomes more refined. As we become more mindful, we act more authentically, as we act more authentically, our minds become clearer, and we can look more deeply into our experience.

Like any structure, a relationship's strength depends on the integrity of its foundation. Since most communication in relationships is sustained through speaking and writing, it is crucial that we nurture honesty in our speech. The Buddha included right speech as a component of his eightfold path. He taught his monks to refrain from untruthful speech, harmful speech, and heedless speech. Practicing satya in the area of speech requires that we give voice only to what we know to be true, without embellishment or exaggeration and without omitting inconvenient details.

I've never been skilled at lying. My attempts to make up stories have been dismal, transparent failures. I haven't developed a pattern of fabrication mainly because there was no payoff. But I certainly remember times when I embellished a story because I felt that the truth was not impressive enough on its own. It's also easy to recall instances when I deliberately left out details that did not support a point I was trying to make.

Most of us have tested these waters. It is a natural part of living and learning in the world. As we move closer to knowing ourselves completely, deception becomes less attractive. When we abide in our authentic self, dishonesty is not an option. Being untruthful eventually becomes impossible.

Often we fudge the truth because we think telling a little white lie will make our lives easier. In reality, telling lies can make our lives very complicated. Have you ever told a lie and then had to make up even more stories to support it? Often one seemingly insignificant untruth can grow into an unwieldy tall tale that becomes increasingly difficult to reverse as we continue to invest more into it. When we invent a story, we don't always remember who we told it to or what we told them. We become saddled with the task of remembering a lot of information that can be difficult to track. It's much easier to recount what actually happened. Telling the truth is simple and clean. When we practice honesty in our speech, clarity and trust imbue our relationships and our lives.

Because ahimsa is the basis of all the yamas, the practice of satya must be grounded in kindness. For example, what do you say when you run into a friend who has just gotten a haircut that you think looks really awful? In the effort to be impeccably honest, do you offer your opinion? Satya does not ask you to be honest in a way that is hurtful. Because satya springs from the ground of ahimsa, it should never be used as a weapon. Instead, look at your friend through the clear eyes of objectivity. Remember that your opinion of her haircut is just that—your opinion. What can you honestly say that will express a positive truth? You might note that the new hairstyle frames your friend's face nicely, or if it's a radical change, you might note that it makes a bold and adventuresome statement. Or perhaps silence is the best policy.

Speech is extremely powerful. It is crucial that we use such a potent resource with care and wisdom. There are many ways that we use speech to cause harm. Sometimes we speak angrily or even violently. Angry and violent speech are a form of abuse and are just as damaging to the recipient as physical abuse.

In his book *The Heart of the Buddha's Teaching*, Thich Nhat Hanh suggests that when we feel the impulse to speak angrily, we instead step back and allow the anger to cool before verbalizing our concerns. When we feel the heat of anger boiling up in us, he suggests that we ask the other person (the object of our anger) if we can continue our conversation in a day or two, when we can speak from a place of greater clarity and kindness. He does not ask us to deny our anger, which can turn its poison back on ourselves. Rather, his suggestion allows us to acknowledge honestly what we are feeling but prevents us from causing further damage by attacking another.

Gossip is another form of harmful speech. When we speak harshly about someone who is not present, we harm that person. The person has no opportunity to offer his or her perspective or to defend against our attacks. Gossip is completely one-sided and rarely acknowledges the viewpoint of its object. We also hurt ourselves, because we are practicing, and therefore cultivating, a pattern of harmful and deceitful speech.

Gossip is harmful because it nurtures negativity. It is deceitful because when we gossip we do not speak our concerns directly to the person who is the subject of our gossip. We may even be kind to this person when we are in her presence, while berating her when her back is turned. This puts us in a state of conflict. One part of us uplifts the person with kindness, while the other part tears her down. The practice of refraining from speaking negatively about someone who is not present is life-affirming. It strengthens the qualities of ahimsa and satya.

Pujari suggests that before we say something, we ask ourselves two questions: Is it true? and Is it useful? In her book *Living Your Yoga*, Judith Hanson Lasater adds the question, Is it nonharming? Many relational traps can be avoided by asking these questions before launching into speech that might be hurtful, untrue, or unnecessary. When I remember to filter my speech through these questions, I speak a lot less and listen a lot more

When I was in college, my friends and I often sat around our in the wee hours of the morning not saying a word. After a while the quiet became too much to bear. Invariably someone—sometimes I—would begin to babble nervously, simply to break the silence. The act of talking just to avoid discomfort was rarely fruitful. The anxiety from which it sprang often added to the awkwardness in the atmosphere. I've since become quite comfortable with silence among friends. The ability to abide in silence with someone bespeaks a deep level of comfort and companionship with that person.

Sutra II.36 says: "When we are firmly established in truthfulness, action accomplishes its desired end." This translation (by Alistair Shearer), along with the following (by Barbara Stoler Miller), forms the basis for my interpretation of this sutra. "When one abides in truthfulness, activity and its fruition are grounded in the truth." Abiding in truthfulness—seeing clearly without the filters of our psychological patterns—allows our actions and their results to be consistent with our true intentions. This speaks to the importance of knowing ourselves. Awareness of our possible blind spots, as well as clarification of our intention, bring the results of our actions into alignment with our deepest truth.

From living mindfully, authenticity arises. It comes from knowing ourselves. Living authentically ensures that we will act with integrity. Sometimes it is difficult to trust that our decisions will bring about fruitful results, especially when we are easily influenced by others' opinions. As we practice satya, living truthfully becomes easier and eventually becomes a habit that replaces old, harmful patterns.

Through deep listening we hear the voice of truth. At first, we may not want to hear what this voice is telling us. Over time, we begin to trust it and to rely on it to guide our lives. Pay attention to your intuition, those feelings from your gut that signal that you might be preparing to use words as weapons or to say something that might not be completely true. What do you hope to accomplish by speaking? As you formulate what you are about to say, ask yourself honestly, Is it true? Is it useful? Is it nonharming? If it is not, continue listening. Listening is the key to contacting satya in yourself. Listen deeply. Speak with care.

Satya in Your Asana Practice

Practicing asana from your deepest integrity requires that you be both mindful and respectful of your body's capabilities. Practicing in integrity requires that you know and respect the truth of this moment's practice. Perhaps last week, or even yesterday, you were able to practice Utthita Trikonasana (Extended Triangle Pose) with your hand resting easily on the floor. Today you can do it only if you bend your trunk and restrict your breathing. Placing a block under your bottom hand would allow you to practice Triangle with integrity.

Practicing asana from the perspective of satya requires that you be mindful, and that you understand that today's practice is not yesterday's practice. Each time you approach asana practice—even those poses you may have done thousands of times—it is the first time you have practiced at this moment in your life.

Can you practice each pose with a beginner's curiosity? This not only allows you to practice with integrity but also keeps your asana practice fresh and interesting.

Reflections

■ Before you speak, notice your intention for what you plan to say. Is your intention simply to add information to the conversation? Is it to demonstrate your superior knowledge of a subject? Ask yourself the three questions: Is what I'm about to say true? Is it useful? Is it nonharming?

■ Notice your listening style. When another person is talking, are you listening to what they are saying or are you formulating your own response as they speak? Resolve to look directly at the person speaking and listen to what they say before you begin planning your response.

■ Practice letting go of gossip. Resolve not to talk about someone who is not present in the room.

■ Note the times when you find yourself wanting to tell only a partial truth by embellishing a story or by leaving out inconvenient details. As a practice, tell stories only if you can do so without exaggerations or omissions.

Asteya: Practicing Abundance 9

S ITTING ATOP a mountain at 8,700 feet, the Last Resort is incomparably gorgeous in the wintertime. Mounds of virgin snow, made blue by the reflection of the indigo sky, blanket the trees, rocks, and cabins. The piercing winter sun creates sparkles in the snow that appear suspended in the air. These multicolored pinpoints of light inspire fairyland imaginings, as they shift and dance with each step. The rarefied mountain air vibrates with the clarity of pure awareness.

Winter also brings logistical complications to the retreat center. When five or six feet of snow cover the ground, the place is accessible only by snowmobile or Snow Cat. The wood-burning stove needs to be fed constantly; its fuel needs to be kept dry during snowstorms. Most of all, until quite recently, water was scarce. The subdivision planners failed to bury the water pipes deep enough to avoid freezing in coldest temperatures, so from October through April the water was turned off completely. (A new, year-round water system has been installed throughout the subdivision.) Residents had to haul their water up the mountain, often by snowmobile, to small holding tanks that pumped this most precious resource into the cabins. When ten extra yogis occupied the center for the winter meditation retreats, all had to be mindful of conservation.

At first, I resented taking sponge baths instead of hot showers. Not flushing the toilets (unless it was absolutely necessary) rankled my sanitized Western sensibilities. Washing and rinsing dishes in a few inches of water seemed ineffective. When I arrived home after a retreat, I would head for the shower immediately. But I noticed that instead of luxuriating in pounding hot water for fifteen minutes, I turned the water off when I wasn't using it. It felt wasteful to leave the water running as I washed dishes. I realized that I really didn't need to flush five gallons of water down the loo every single time I used it.

The retreat had taught me about cooperation. I was inspired by the small sacrifices each yogi made on the retreat in order to ensure that there was enough water for everyone. I realized on a profound level that we all share resources on this planet. While we might wonder whether our singular acts of conservation actually make a difference in this world, when we understand our deep connection with all other beings it becomes difficult to let our precious and finite resources go to waste simply because it might be inconvenient to turn off a light or a water faucet.

The third of the yamas is *asteya*. Literally translated as "nonstealing," asteya asks that we take only what is offered and use only what we need. Practicing asteya teaches us about interconnectedness in the same way that practicing ahimsa and satya do. Our actions do have repercussions, some that we see, many that we do not. When we take what is not offered, we are showing a lack of respect for others and the resources they have saved for themselves. When we take more than we need, we leave less for all other beings who share the planet's resources.

Asteya can be practiced in the realms of material resources, intellectual material, and time and energy. Material resources include all the worldly matter we need to survive—food, water, shelter—and those things we don't necessarily need but that make life more enjoyable—cars, phones, clothing, books, music, and so on. Intellectual material includes ideas and concepts. Respect for others' personal boundaries allows us to practice asteya in the realms of time and energy.

Years ago, I sometimes sampled items in the bulk bins at the natural foods store. While I'm certain even now that the store could easily absorb the loss of an occasional chocolate-covered almond or fig bar, as I began practicing mindfulness I realized that the size or importance of what I so freely pilfered was not the issue. I saw that in helping myself to items not offered I was cultivating a habit of stealing. Each time I sampled some new item, I thought less and less about the repercussions of my actions. Each instance reinforced the idea that it was okay to take something that had not been freely offered. Ultimately this was not a habit I wanted to cultivate.

Respect for others' time and energy is another manifestation of asteya. I have observed myself having long phone conversations with old friends, nudging our interactions along, simply because I wanted or needed connection. Sometimes the other person expresses an interest in ending the conversation, but I hang on and keep it going. This is taking advantage of another's time when she is too polite to assert her needs. I have also been on the receiving end of this kind of interaction because I am not always skilled at asserting my own boundaries.

A simple solution for avoiding being on either end of this form of time and energy overconsumption is to set the ground rules before the conversation begins. When we initiate a conversation, we can ask at the outset if the other person has time to talk. When someone else contacts us, we can state before the conversation gains momentum that while we can't talk now, perhaps there's another time that would work for both of us.

The desire to take from someone else or to consume more than we need is based in a feeling of lack, a sense that we do not have all that we need in this moment. It is this feeling of deficiency that allows us to justify overconsumption. After all, if we don't take what we can right now, someone else might grab it, and then there will be less for us. A feeling of lack, which sometimes is accompanied by a sense of entitlement, can seem to justify a desire to take something that clearly belongs to someone else.

On retreats at the Last Resort, we are asked to refine our asteya practice to the point where we do not even sample someone else's shampoo in the bathrooms that we share. This creates an environment of trust. Even though we all share a relatively small space, participants feel completely comfortable leaving doors unlocked and open, with our possessions in full view.

Sutra II.37 (Miller) says: "When one abjures stealing, jewels shower down." When we respect others' resources, they can feel free to offer us their gifts of time, energy, and material goods because they trust that we will not take advantage of their generosity.

Asteya is often translated as "honesty" or "integrity" as well as "nonstealing." Integrity inspires trust. When we are honest in our dealings with people, they naturally want to interact with us. If we act with integrity in our business dealings, our business thrives. If we are trustworthy as friends, we enjoy an abundance of friendships.

Mindfulness helps us see our inherent wholeness. When we are mindful, we see that nothing is lacking in this moment, that we are complete as we are. We gain entry into the awareness that binds us all. As a result, we become less self-centered and therefore less likely to take more than we need. When we feel complete as we are and connected to the web of life, we realize that sharing in itself is abundance.

Asteya in Your Asana Practice

I injured myself only once in asana practice. It happened when another teacher told me that I wasn't doing a proper Salamba Sirsasana (Headstand) because my weight was not equally balanced between my head and my arms. Because I'd previously suffered a whiplash injury, I relied on my arm strength to hold me up. Feeling inadequate in the face of the other teacher's superior pose, I let my head bear as much weight as my arms. After all, it was important that I be as "advanced" in my pose as she was. Almost immediately, I felt a painful stabbing in my neck and shoulder that reignited my whiplash injury. Six months of chiropractic treatment and six months of doing absolutely no Headstands finally cured the injury.

Comparing ourselves to others is no more helpful in asana practice than it is in the rest of our lives. My father was extremely flexible, a gymnast who competed nationally. I inherited his flexibility, making many asanas quite easy for me. However, until I began practicing standing poses, I never knew how little strength I had developed. Others in the class accomplished the standing poses much more easily.

We all come into the world with genetic traits that either help or hinder our performance of asanas. In addition, we spend many years developing habits of posture or body carriage that affect how we practice. Coveting or resenting someone else's superior-looking postures does not serve us. Nor does thinking less of someone whose poses do not rise to the level of ours. The practice is about discovering our unique patterns, bolstering those that affect us positively, and repatterning those that do not serve us. Remember that your practice is entirely yours. Celebrate others' unique abilities as well as your own.

Reflections

- Do you leave lights on in unoccupied rooms? Do you leave the TV on while no one is watching it? Do you run the water while shaving, brushing your teeth, or doing the dishes? Do you leave your cell phone charger plugged in when you're not using it?[1] Do you take unnecessary trips in your car? Consider how you might save gas by combining errands. Become mindful of your consumption habits. Teach your kids about conservation, and help them develop conscious conservation practices that they can carry throughout their lives.

- When you want to talk with friends, colleagues, or family members, especially if the conversation promises to be involved, first ask if they have time. If not, schedule a time when you can converse without having to think about time constraints.

- Give credit where it is due. Even if you are not legally bound to attribute someone's ideas or quotes, give them credit, even in ordinary, friendly conversation. This helps you develop appreciation for your network of support.

---

1. According to www.futureforests.com, in the UK only 5 percent of the power used by cell phone chargers goes to powering phones. The rest is used when the charger is plugged in and switched on but not in use. That's 50,000 tons of CO_2 that could be eliminated in the UK alone, just by unplugging cell phone chargers.

Brahmacharya: 10
Caring for Our Creative Energy

I'S MID-APRIL as I begin this chapter. Each day as I survey my garden, I see new growth, new life. The fruit trees in my backyard are laden with blossoms. Splashy, rainbow-hued tulips usher me along my front sidewalk. The tiny perennials I welcomed to my front yard last fall are thriving. The very air feels redolent with abundant life.

As I sit at my computer, contemplating how to begin this chapter of the yamas, I happen to glance upward at my office window. There I see two box elder bugs, a species that feeds on the seedpods of female box elder trees. The bugs are crawling along my windowsill, linked rear end to rear end, in their mating posture. This familiar springtime vignette reminds me that divine creative energy exists always, in every living thing: in the box elder bugs' breeding ritual, the seed pods on which they feed, and the burgeoning plant life in my yard.

Creative, sexual energy is the divine force that animates every living thing. Mammals conceive by uniting egg and sperm. The wind scatters seeds and pollen to create new plant growth. Everything that is alive on this earth exists because of sexual energy. It is the seed from which all creative pursuits begin.

Creative energy resides within us. We can express this force in many positive ways, by conceiving and nurturing children or pursuing artistic endeavors, or by channeling its power into whatever moves us. We also can express this energy in negative ways, by using our sexuality to manipulate another or by giving life to any behavior that causes harm to others or to ourselves.

Brahmacharya, the fourth yama, asks us to care for and express sexual energy in ways that sustain our planet and ourselves. While it is often interpreted as celibacy or, more moderately, wise use of our sexuality, Donna Farhi, in her book *Yoga Mind, Body and Spirit*, suggests that brahmacharya means "merging with the one." Brahmacharya expresses union with the energy that produces life in all its forms. We can give birth to new human beings, to creative endeavors of all kinds, and to thoughts and dreams.

The wide range of interpretations offered by sutra translators is a testament to brahmacharya's flexible, and sometimes controversial, meaning. Alistair Shearer translates Sutra II.38 as: "When we are firmly established in chastity, subtle potency is generated." Barbara Stoler Miller's translation is similar: "When one observes celibacy, heroic energy accrues." T. K. V. Desikachar suggests a wider interpretation: "At its best, moderation produces the highest individual vitality." Kofi Busia's translation mirrors Farhi's concept of merging with the one. He writes, "Through communion with God, one becomes truly strong." While the range of interpretation for the first phrase of this sutra is rather wide, all these translations agree in their declarations that we accrue strength and vitality by caring for our divine sexual energy.

In a monastic setting, brahmacharya is a practice of abstention. Rather than being dispersed through sexual activity, creative energies are channeled into the pursuit of awakening. The practice of celibacy can be a source of happiness and fulfillment when it is undertaken voluntarily, in contrast to when it is imposed upon us by an outer or inner mandate.

Too often, sexual abstention is dictated by a spiritual leader or doctrine and is maintained by feelings of guilt or self-righteousness. This manifestation of brahmacharya frequently implodes, because forced suppression is not a balanced or respectful way to control such a powerful energy.

It is not unusual for the very guru who commands that his disciples abstain from sexual activity to be revealed as having participated in indiscretions of his own. And forced celibacy squashes the infinite energy it is supposed to generate. While we might take a temporary vow of celibacy during a meditation retreat, most of us living in twenty-first-century America interpret brahmacharya more moderately. Most yogis in this culture live as householders. Whether or not we choose to use our sexual energy to create families, many of us choose to invest at least some of this energy into our primary relationships. The practice for those of us living in the secular world is about learning to use our sexuality to generate healthy connection, a merging of the divine at the core of our beloved and ourselves.

In Western culture, the pendulum of sexual belief swings from one extreme to the other. Much religious doctrine teaches that sexuality is immoral, one of the seven deadly sins. On the other end of the pendulum swing, popular culture—from television programs and commercials to pop music and movies—portrays sex as the forbidden fruit that we all secretly want more than anything, the be-all and end-all that will make us happy. This creates a powerful confusion and has led to a great deal of abuse of sexual energy. So I especially like Desikachar's use of the word "moderation" for this sutra. I see brahmacharya as a commitment to using sexual energy wisely, neither suppressing it nor overindulging.

Wise use of sexual energy means neither denying nor judging our desires and also not becoming enslaved by our biology. This is a delicate process. When we suppress desire, we deny the force of life, and it comes back in unpredictable and harmful ways. On the other hand, when we overindulge this energy, using it wantonly and unconsciously, we deplete ourselves. We harm our partners when we use them simply to fulfill our desires. Brahmacharya, like all the yamas, is rooted in ahimsa. Can we share our creative energy in a way that is nourishing for everyone involved?

Most of us have experienced the staggering range of emotions that accompanies romantic relationships. When a relationship is going well, we feel optimistic, fulfilled, elated. After a breakup, or when we're disappointed with a relationship, we feel sadness, resentment, jealousy, even downright hatred. These peaks and valleys are a testament to the power of sexual energy. When we are caught in these all-consuming highs and lows, it is helpful to be mindful of what we feel and to look at how we project our own emotions onto the other.

In his book *We*, Robert Johnson explains romantic love as the projection of divine qualities onto the human object of our fancy. He suggests that in the era when romantic love became fashionable, humanity simply shifted its spiritual ardor from gods to lovers. Humans hold a deep desire to merge with the divine. In the age of reason, Western culture gave up its worship of unseen entities, only to project godlike qualities onto fallible human beings. The essential desire to merge was transferred to idealized men and women.

If Johnson's theory is valid, it's no wonder that we so often feel resentful and betrayed when our ideal lover begins to show his or her human qualities. The fall of a god or goddess is not a pretty sight, even if their divinity existed only in our heads. However, according to this model, healthy union also can be seen as an expression of merging with the divine: that divine energy that is the essential substance of our being.

I've come to understand that the wise expression of sexual energy can happen in a number of ways, within a committed relationship or in the context of a more casual connection. How a relationship looks is not as important as the intention we bring to it. Knowing, as we do from experience, the power our sexuality has to create great happiness or profound sadness can guide us in offering our energy appropriately.

This means we share our sexuality only with consenting adults. Forcing our sexuality onto an unwilling partner is an act of violence. Brahmacharya asks that we honor our commitments if we are involved in an exclusive relationship. We must also honor the relationships of others and not compromise them by becoming involved with people who are committed to another.

We must take care not to abuse positions of authority, such as supervisory, therapeutic, or teaching positions, to manipulate employees, clients, or students into sexual affairs. As a yoga teacher, I am quite familiar with the occasional student's tendency to project superhuman qualities onto me. Because of my own ego habit of underplaying my talents and abilities, I have not been seduced into believing these projections—at least not for very long—or exploiting the student–teacher relationship for personal gain. After many years of practicing mindfulness, I am well aware of my own very ordinary nature, with its panoply of positive attributes and shortcomings. Like my students, I am simply human—nothing more, nothing less.

However, it is easy to understand how a teacher can begin to believe students' unrealistic projections. Receiving praise feels wonderful. And we are all essentially divine after all. The problem comes when a teacher and student agree, either consciously or unconsciously, that the former is more divine than the latter. This uneven relationship sets the ground for potential abuse. It is the teacher's responsibility to maintain boundaries if the urge to enter into a romantic involvement becomes strong. On the other hand, if it seems that there is potential for a healthy and fruitful pairing between a student and teacher, it may be best that the student find another teacher, so that both parties can stand as equals.

How can we find balance in our practice of brahmacharya? On the sexual plane, we can begin by examining the motivations for expressing our sexuality. Are we engaging in sexual activity simply to fulfill our own needs or desires, or is there an intention to share a profound union with the other? Do we engage in sexual connections in order to feel loved, or in order to feel powerful? With so much potential woven into the fabric of sexuality, can we begin to consider our modes of expression more carefully?

If we choose celibacy as a voluntary practice, or if we are alone, how can we use our energy wisely? Since sexual energy is the basis for all creative energy, there are myriad ways to express it. Artists often go on a "sexual fast" while they are focusing on a major project, in order to channel their creativity into their artistic pursuits. Spiritual practitioners such as Mother Teresa have invested their life energy into helping others. Householders give their energy to creating stable, healthy families, or they might give themselves to their work. Bodhisattvas dedicate their energy to awakening. There is no end to the ways we can put this energy to positive effect in the world, whether or not we are expressing it sexually.

This energy is sacred. It is infinitely powerful. We can use it to give birth to actions that nourish our world or destroy it. Use it with joyful moderation. Consider its grounding in ahimsa. Merge with the divine—in yourself, in the person you love, and in all creation.

Brahmacharya in Your Asana Practice

Do you ever find yourself reflecting on your day or planning for some future commitment while you practice your forward bends? This is an effective way to fritter away your essential energy. Asana practice provides an exquisite avenue to care for, channel, and even increase the flow of your divine life force. Practicing with the mind fully, inquisitively engaged in the ever-changing present sensations of asana practice conserves and reinvests our energy into ourselves. Practicing asana while thinking about something completely unrelated dissipates our vital energy and squanders the potential of asana practice.

While we might think of asana as the picture-perfect, static poses captured in so many books and magazines, asana is actually a process that begins with our intention to place our bodies in a particular position. We can practice brahmacharya by becoming mindful of the entire process—from our initial intention through each incremental micromovement along the way to manifestation of the formal asana, to all the subtle movements that occur as we hold an asana, and to those movements that take us back to center. Practicing in this way not only conserves and builds our vital energy, it makes for a satisfying and informative practice moment to moment.

In practicing brahmacharya in asana, it is also helpful to remember that greater effort does not necessarily produce greater results. Be aware of how you might be forcing effort in a pose. Engage your entire body equally.

When you practice, simply practice. Set aside the thoughts and plans that vie for your attention. Most assuredly, they will be readily available to you when you finish your practice. Invest yourself entirely in all stages of each asana.

Reflections

- Consider the possible ways in which you squander your creative/sexual energy. How can you conserve this energy so that you can invest it in the ways you choose?

- Examine your motivations for engaging in sexual intimacy. When you think about partnering sexually, is it with your own pleasure or the other person's pleasure in mind? Does sexuality feel like a need or a compulsion? Or does its attraction lie in sharing a bit of your divine energy with another? Reflect on ways you can find a balance between suppressing this energy and overindulging.

Aparigraha: 11
The Freedom of Letting Go

IN 2003, an acupuncturist named Denise closed her thriving Salt Lake City clinic and opened a restaurant based on a bold and compassionate vision. One World Café is a tiny buffet-style restaurant in the heart of the city. Its motto is "Everybody Eats." Customers are encouraged to choose only as much as they can eat to cut down on waste. The food is organically grown and cooked fresh each day. Food left over at the day's end is donated to the homeless. Denise pays employees a living wage. There is no set price for a meal. Customers contribute whatever they can afford.

You might expect that One World Café would quickly go the way of so many conventional restaurants and collapse within a short time. But on the contrary, the café has been a great success. Denise says that the outpouring of generosity from the community has been overwhelming. One landowner offered her a valuable city block of open space to plant an organic garden. A master gardener stepped forward to oversee the project—for free. Grateful customers have donated dishes and silverware and have volunteered their time and energy to help out in various ways. One customer gave Denise a car. So out of the ordinary is the concept of trust and generosity in business that local and national media have sought out Denise to honor her and her vision. One World Café has been featured in *People* magazine and on National Public Radio (NPR).

Denise took a great risk in letting go of her acupuncture practice. As stable and lucrative as it was, her business no longer inspired her. She felt called to help feed the hungry, and her vision has grown and begun to send out tentacles to other cities. In following her heart's calling, Denise fashioned a life for herself that is fulfilling, rich with appreciation, and always new. She has experienced the abundance of generosity and the freedom of letting go.

When Sogyal Rinpoche, author of *The Tibetan Book of Living and Dying*, spoke in Salt Lake City, he made a statement that has stayed with me. He said, "Freedom does not come from acquisition. It comes from letting go." In the same way that the rotten vegetables in our refrigerator occupy space that could be filled with fresh, vital foods, the habits we grasp onto for security stultify us. We can't move forward in our lives when we cling to the past. When we set our habits, our beliefs, and our ways of living in concrete, we become imprisoned by them. Letting go of what is no longer appropriate in our lives releases us to all possibilities.

The fifth yama is *aparigraha*, nonattachment. Aparigraha is also sometimes translated as "nongreed" or "nongrasping." Nonattachment is one of the basic tenets of Buddhist practice. The Buddha considered attachment to be a root cause of suffering. Because all things are impermanent, seeking security by holding on to things that will, by their very nature, always go away creates pain and suffering. How many possessions, practices, jobs, people, animals, relationships, and even identities have you held for a time and then let go? The number is truly staggering for all of us.

Sometimes we do not choose to let go; the circumstances of our lives often dictate that we must. Relationships dissolve. Once-inspiring careers become stagnant, and we are moved to create something new. Friends and relatives come and go; they move away or pass away. Our bodies change as we age. Sometimes disease dictates that we change our lives radically.

When we experience a loss, or when it comes time to let go of something we hold dear, it is natural to mourn. It is nearly impossible not to wonder how much easier or better our lives might be if our circumstances could continue as usual. But the reality of living is that our lives change constantly. Without continuous change, it would be impossible to grow. It is letting go of the old, the things we no longer need, that makes room in our lives for whatever is to come.

Our lives are a continuum of receiving and releasing, receiving and releasing. Thousands of times each day, our bodies naturally draw in and release the breath. When we inhale, we receive the vital oxygen that enlivens the cells of our bodies. When we exhale, we expel toxic waste in the form of carbon dioxide. What would happen to our bodies if we only inhaled or held one breath all day? What if we chose only to accumulate and never to let go?

The Buddha found that happiness is available to everyone when we let go of searching for it in those things that are not permanent. When we rely on our bodies, our careers, our friends and family to make us happy and secure, we set ourselves up to suffer. Ultimately all must be released.

Early in my asana study, I practiced intensely and attained the strength, flexibility, and technique required to accomplish many of the most advanced asanas. More than two decades later, even though I might fondly remember those times of physical accomplishment, would I really want to return there? What I have let go in terms of extreme practice has made room for a more mature, more satisfying awareness of the subtle energies that govern my body's essential vitality. As a result, my practice has gained integrity, and my body has become stronger and more balanced.

As we live and grow, our understanding becomes more refined. Out of the process of continual drawing in and letting go, compassion and wisdom grow. Kofi Busia's translation of Sutra II.39 on aparigraha says, "Knowledge of the beginning and end of all past and present being comes through the continued correct practice of not holding on to things." As we come to peace with the reality of constant change, wisdom grows. We understand that each forward step on life's path requires us to let go of the previous step. The process of living rests in the delicate balance between the death of the old and the birth of the new.

You can easily see the constant flow of impermanent phenomena by looking at your own mind. Sit quietly and watch your thoughts. The myriad sensations that come and go, within even a few minutes, is quite astounding. When we can come to peace with the flow of activity in our own minds, we can begin to relax into the rhythm of change that is the only constant in our lives.

How can we practice aparigraha? If a loss forces us to let go, we can reflect on how we might best welcome the changes we must make. We can take advantage of the opportunity to bring something new into our lives. Sometimes, like Denise, we see that a situation or relationship no longer feeds us, and we make the choice to let go and begin something new.

Practicing generosity is a powerful and pleasurable way to develop aparigraha. Generosity is the first of the Buddha's ten *paramitas*, the qualities of mind and heart of a bodhisattva. He encouraged his monks to cultivate generosity before all else. In a moment of giving, generosity creates happiness for the giver and the receiver. Giving also brings happiness when we reflect on a prior act of generosity, whether we are on the giving or receiving side. Finally, each time we share, we cultivate and strengthen the habit of giving.

Pujari advises his students to always follow through when the urge to give arises. So many times I've felt the exhilaration of a generous intention, then watched glumly as I talked myself out of it. In practicing this resolve, I've found that I hear almost instantly from the voices that proclaim my own lack. These voices remind me that I might someday need the object to be given, or that I can't possibly afford to share. While it might be wise to consider my resources, now when the impulse to give comes up I always follow it in some way. I have never regretted it later.

There are many ways to develop generosity. Buy a gift or share a meal. Donate some of your possessions to a friend in need or to a charity. Offer some of your time and energy, perhaps by volunteering for a nonprofit group or serving at a shelter. Be available to the people in your life. Make a phone call to a distant friend. Write an old-fashioned longhand letter. The next time a friend wants to tell you a story or ask your advice, really listen, without an agenda. An act of generosity doesn't have to be grandiose to bring happiness.

Happiness comes from enjoying your life right now. When you live mindfully, even the most mundane tasks of your daily routine can be joyful. When you give your complete attention to the present realities of your life, there is no residue left to cling to when it is time to let go and move on. Being fully present with your daily process of receiving and releasing brings the equanimity that allows you to flow with the cycles of constant change.

Aparigraha in Your Asana Practice

Over the years, I have observed myself giving less than 100 percent to my asana practice, simply because I feared I would use up my energy and feel tired later. The truth is, when I give all of my physical, mental, and emotional energies to my practice, I feel fulfilled afterward, much more so than when I hold back. Even my experience of Savasana (Relaxation Pose) is more satisfying and profound when I pour myself completely into it. There is no leftover residue of unspent energy to make my mind and body restless.

Be generous with your effort when you practice. Each asana gives back the amount of energy that we invest into it. Energy is not finite; you gain in exact proportion to what you give. This of course applies not only to asana practice but to whatever you choose to do. Invest yourself totally in all your life practices. Leave nothing behind.

Reflections

- Practice generosity. When the urge to give arises, follow it.

- Reflect on the many identities you have constructed and then discarded when they no longer felt appropriate. Are there any ways in which you define yourself now that no longer serve you? What habits—physical, mental, or emotional—are you ready to release? In the past when you released worn out habits or beliefs, what happened? How did you grow from your many experiences of letting go? It is possible to meet the multitude of let-go experiences still to come with a sense of joy and adventure. Revisit this practice several times a year.

- Cultivate generosity in your asana practice. Begin each session by assessing what is feasible for your practice today. What time is available? What kind of energy are you bringing to practice today? Is your energy abundant or lacking? What's going on in your body? Are there certain areas that need extra attention? Practice asana with respect for what is possible for you each day.

The Second Limb
Niyama: Conscious Everyday Living 12

M Y VERY FIRST asana class registered an unexpected blow to my ego. Before the class I thought of myself as extraordinarily flexible, based on memories of the loosely knit, unwieldy, ten-year-old body I enjoyed when I studied ballet as a child. At twenty-six, however, after years of hiking and biking, touching my toes was but a dream. When I was young, I loved to make people gasp at my ability to fall into side splits, then bend forward flat-backed and rest my chin on the floor. Now the floor was hopelessly out of reach. And falling into side splits surely would have caused grave injury. I felt terribly humbled as we moved through the asana routine.

As difficult as my newly discovered stiffness was to digest, I felt oddly at peace and rejuvenated after being led through the guided relaxation at the end of class. As I turned on my car to return home, a familiar rock song exploded from the radio. I may as well have been punched in the face. Immediately I turned down the volume. Not good enough. I began dialing through the stations. As the pointer moved across the radio's face, all amplified music and commentary felt harsh and invasive. It was not until I reached NPR, broadcasting Beethoven's Symphony no. 1, that the music I heard harmonized with the state of my nervous system.

I didn't realize it then, but I was already beginning the process of shifting my daily habits to align with what would become a lifelong commitment to yoga. Though this thought did not cross my mind at the time, I was beginning to realize that there are some things we do in the course of our days that support the cultivation of yoga—the settling of the mind into silence—and others that do not. (For the record, yoga practice did not forever condemn me to listening only to quiet music. I still joyously attend an annual four-day orgy of amplified music at the Telluride Bluegrass Festival, as well as concerts of many genres throughout the year. During and after practice, however, I prefer silence.)

Patanjali's Yoga Sutras list five daily practices, called niyamas, which taken together form a solid, fertile foundation in which to cultivate the settled mind. The niyamas are: purity; cultivation of contentment; simplicity, discipline, or enthusiasm; self-study and the study of sacred literature; and surrender to grace.

In T. K. V. Desikachar's sutra translation, he describes the yamas as "our attitudes towards our environment" and the niyamas as "our attitudes towards ourselves." In her book *Yoga Mind, Body and Spirit*, Donna Farhi titles the section addressing the niyamas "codes for living soulfully." I see the niyamas as daily practices that, when undertaken with intention, clear a path for spiritual evolution.

The niyamas are practices that help us clean and cultivate our physical, mental, and emotional palates. When we tend a garden by feeding and watering the plants we wish to cultivate and weeding out those that compete for nutrients in the soil, our chosen plants grow strong and healthy. In the same way, when we cultivate the niyamas, we clear our environments as well as our bodies and minds of those qualities that create agitation, while we strengthen those qualities that uncover our essential quiet mind.

Previous to my first yoga retreat at the Last Resort, I had no idea that yoga extended beyond my asana practice. Observing Pujari and Abhilasha living a yogic life, and experiencing a week devoted entirely to practice, gave me a new understanding of yoga. In addition to two daily sessions of intense asana, we practiced pranayama and meditation and took invigorating hikes in the surrounding mountains. Rather than being a how-to course on the minutiae of correct asana practice, the retreat focused on the process of living a yogic life. We devoted retreat time to real-life subjects such as right livelihood and right relationship. Most days included a class with Abhilasha on natural nutrition and the necessity of nourishing the body in order to maintain mental equilibrium.

I returned home from the retreat inspired and somewhat overwhelmed by the vast scope of what I now understood to be the yogic life. As good as asana practice made me feel, performing poses for an hour a day and then stowing my mat and sleepwalking through the rest of my life was no longer an option. I had to ask myself how, as a city dweller with a full-time job, I could let my practice infiltrate my life so the whole thing became an expression of yoga. I found out that the most practical answer to this question is: gradually. Patience is a necessity. Changing ingrained habits requires commitment. It also requires compassion. Whipping oneself into living a yogic life is impossible.

In one nutrition class, Pujari and Abhilasha suggested setting aside one day each month as "goop day." On that day you get to eat a corn dog, a chocolate bar, or a pizza with extra everything—joyfully, without guilt or self-judgment. This outlet tends to defuse the temptation to indulge at other times and often takes a bit of the sheen off your forbidden fruit. For many of us, prohibition often renders something more attractive than it would be otherwise. Removing the glamour lessens the desire.

The occasional goop day reminds us that what's most important is not what we do once in a while but what we do day to day. Those habits we cultivate every day become the substance of who we are. When our daily practices are aimed at promoting a settled mind, we can step off our path once in a while and not be thrown out of balance. With the niyamas as our foundation, we can sustain the occasional physical, mental, or emotional goop day (or goop week) without losing our center.

Like the yamas, the niyamas are not intended to be unbending law. As with anything we choose to practice, over time our relationship with the niyamas will evolve. How we express the niyamas ten years from now may bear little resemblance to how our practice looks today. Remaining open to the myriad ways of interpreting the niyamas to fit our individual journeys allows the practice to stay vital.

Along with the yamas and asana, the niyamas are among the first practices traditionally given to aspiring yogis. As with the yamas, I have found it helpful to focus on one niyama at a time for as long as it takes for me to integrate it and its effects. Like anything to which we apply ourselves, niyama practice eventually becomes effortless. Practice becomes unnecessary, as these qualities become the ground on which we live and grow.

Reflections

■ Commit to practicing one niyama for a specified period of time—for a month, several months, or a year. At the end of that time, reflect on what you've learned and how your life has changed. You may want to record your intentions in a journal and check in with it every so often during the month or year to see if and how you'd like to modify your practice. Decide whether this niyama needs continued attention or whether it has become sufficiently integrated that you'd like to begin practicing another one.

■ Choose one day each week or month to suspend your niyama practice. Reflect on any positive or negative results. If you are generally a very disciplined person, note how a day of being lax affects you. Conversely if you are generally not disciplined, note the effects of a day deliberately without discipline.

Saucha: Cultivating Purity 13

THERE WERE MANY things I was not prepared for when I sat my first vipassana retreat in 1988. I could not have imagined the profound satisfaction of experiencing, even for a few moments, a mind that was temporarily cleared of its usual agitations. I also could not have imagined how my brief encounter with mental clarity would alter my daily life when I returned home.

While I had not previously been a pathological collector of clutter, I have a certain threshold for disorder in my home. Piles of unpaid bills, magazines, books and records, as well as a plethora of knickknacks covered most of the horizontal surfaces in my house. Mostly the piles of paper did not bother me, as long as they were stacked and not slumping too far over their boundaries.

When I returned from retreat, however, the clutter in my house made me feel claustrophobic. With my mind relatively clear of its usual disorder, I could no longer tolerate the chaos in my environment. It was hard for me to feel settled when my home was in confusion. Clearing the clutter in my environment became a daily practice that proved to be an invaluable support for my clarity of mind. I have consistently found that I can accomplish much more and with greater efficiency if my own (literal) house is in order.

And so began the intentional practice of *saucha*, the first niyama, starting with clearing my physical surroundings. I no longer needed to fill my space with objects that were not useful, and in the process I began to understand the exhilaration of letting go (which in turn supported my fledgling practice of aparigraha). Saucha is the practice of cleanliness or purity. This applies not only to our physical environment and appearance but also to what we take into our bodies and minds.

When I began attending asana classes, I was drinking alcohol only on rare occasions. Still, I remember having a few beers one evening and attending an asana class the next day. I was surprised to find that my body felt weak during practice. I trembled in poses that had been effortless two days before. After sweating and shaking through most of the class, I realized that alcohol was a toxin for my body. The incipient refinement of awareness that asana practice had wrought in those first few months helped me see this for the first time. At that point, the choice to imbibe or not became clear. On special occasions, when I choose to join friends in celebrating with a glass of wine, I enjoy the taste and friendly communion and accept that my body will take a day to return to balance.

Over the years, the ways I practice saucha have become subtler. My body feels much more balanced and calm when I eat simple, whole foods—with only the occasional foray into rich, spicy meals or sweet indulgences. I have also become acutely aware of mental pollution. While I love watching unusual films, I find that I'd rather not see movies that are extremely violent or overly negative. Violent images tend to stay with me long after I leave the theater. They feel mentally and emotionally toxic, not at all conducive to a quiet mind. At least some of the time, I can choose what to plant in my mind. When I can choose, I try not to take in images of violence.

Saucha can also be practiced in relationships. Over the years, I have found myself letting go of those friendships that sustain themselves through unpleasant habits, such as gossip or sarcasm. When I can't minimize my tendency to fall into these patterns in a relationship, I choose to minimize contact with that person. Surrounding yourself with positive and kind people is a powerful way to practice saucha. Along with the buddha (the embodiment of awakening) and the dharma (the truth), sangha—the community of like-minded people—is one of the three jewels that support Buddhist practice. Our daily relationships influence our lives much more than those that we visit only occasionally.

Despite the fact that I have given up many of the things considered pleasurable in twenty-first-century America, I don't feel deprived. As my diet has gradually become cleaner and simpler, my palate has become more sensitive. I no longer need aggressively flavored foods to register enjoyment. The sweet taste of a homegrown tomato is every bit as complex and interesting to me as the most perfectly prepared gourmet entrée.

Some of the translations of Sutra II.40, the first of two sutras that discuss saucha, have been a bit troubling to me. While the interpretations aim to extol the virtues and benefits of practicing saucha, I'm not so sure most people would find the listed benefits palatable. For example, Barbara Stoler Miller translates this sutra: "Aversion to one's own body and avoidance of contact with others comes from bodily purification." Swami Venkatesananda's translation says, "The habit of cleanliness, if it is not mechanical and ritualistic but intelligent with an understanding of the nature of the decaying physical organism, reveals the impure nature of the physical body: and, there arises disgust for the body and a disinclination for contact with those of others." In a culture where we are already taught to feel aversion to our bodies, particularly the perceived imperfections of their outermost layers, I'm disinclined to offer these ideas as an optimal interpretation for Western yogis.

In his book *Enlightenment: The Yoga Sutras of Patanjali*, author MSI comments on this view of Sutra II.40. While he considers translations such as the above to be valid in a literal sense, and appropriate for those who choose to practice renunciation, he states, "that kind of feeling about bodies is not the result of enlightenment but only the result of straining to be enlightened." He explains saucha as a practice that protects us not from simple contact with others' bodies but from "their diseases as well as their violence of thoughts, words and actions." The natural by-product of saucha, he says, is physical security and invincibility. Practicing saucha creates a field of purity in our body–mind that is able to absorb the impurities visited upon it without being contaminated by them. Like all the niyamas, the continued practice of saucha creates an overall condition of clarity that resists impurity.

T. K. V. Desikachar provides the widest and most inspiring view. His translation states, "When cleanliness is developed it reveals what needs to be constantly maintained and what is eternally clean. What decays is the external. What does not is deep within us." He explains his translation thus: "Our overconcern with and attachment to outward things, which is both transient and superficial, is reduced." He is referring to the distinction between the impermanence and insubstantiality of the body–mind and pure awareness, which exists always.

In Buddhist thought, the end of attachment characterizes the highest stage of enlightenment. So the practice of saucha lends support to our practice of aparigraha and paves the way for the practice of all the other limbs of yoga and indeed to our ultimate freedom. Sutra II.41, which states the result of practicing saucha, bears this out. Alistair Shearer suggests this in his translation of this sutra: "Purity of mind, cheerfulness, mastery of the senses, one-pointedness, and readiness for Self-realization follow."

In the same way that ahimsa forms the foundation of all the yamas, saucha forms the foundation of all the niyamas. As our minds and bodies become clearer, the practices that follow become easier. Before I plant my vegetable garden each year, I must clear out all the leftover dead plants from the previous season. I start each new season with soil that is freshly turned, completely empty of last year's plants, and ready to receive and nourish the next generation. Look at your environment and your physical, mental, and emotional habits. Which of these habits feel like clutter? Begin, one step at a time, letting go of those practices and relationships that obscure your essential purity.

Saucha in Your Asana Practice

Saucha has many applications in asana practice. The first and most obvious is to come to your yoga mat with a clean and well-tended body. When the body is clear of impurities, there are fewer obstacles to obstruct the movement of energy. The same is true for your yoga space. Whether you are in a class or at home, when your props are haphazardly strewn about or your space is in general disarray, the energy in the room moves in a disorderly and agitated fashion. Take time to clean your body and clear your space before you practice.

In almost every evening class I teach, at least one student enters the room in a frenzy—relieved to be in class, but harried from a stressful day. Often it can take half the class for the nervous agitation in this person's body to dissipate. For that reason, I begin each class with a short, five- to ten-minute sitting meditation. This is a time when students can set aside their to-do lists or memories of the things that created such agitation and focus their intention on replenishing their own energies. This period of quiet cleanses the mental palate and allows the students to begin their practice with quieter, less cluttered minds.

When you practice, set aside a few minutes to sit silently. When remnants of your day or plans for the rest of your day arise, set them aside. Give your to-do list a rest. It will be there when you finish. Asana practice is your time to take care of yourself.

Reflections

■ Take a look at your storage space. Is your closet overcrowded with stuff you haven't used in a long time? Old items that you no longer need or want drain your energy. Because I like clothes, my closet can get packed in a very short time if I'm not careful. I've resolved to consider whether to buy that sweater or scarf in the first place. I ask myself how and when I will wear it and what it will go with. If I decide that I still want it, I get rid of something I haven't worn in a while to make space for it. I especially enjoy offering clothing to friends. It's fun to see others giving a once-beloved item new life!

Santosha: 14
Awakening Contentment

S EVERAL TIMES each year, I visit my attic and closets looking for items to give away. While performing this ritual a while back, I came upon an old suitcase—a huge, 1960s-style, navy blue hard shell grip (as my grandma called them), lined in satiny light-blue fabric with little gathered pouches along the sides for small valuables. I marveled at the quaintness of its design and the fact that ergonomically incorrect behemoths such as this have all but disappeared from use.

As I looked at its broad surface, I remembered that this suitcase had at one time performed a crucial function in my daily life. For about six months in 1980 it served as a dining table. We brought no furniture with us when we moved out West, and having no money to buy a kitchen table, my husband and I enjoyed many a fine dinner on the suitcase's expanse. On special occasions we would cover it with a fancy scarf and add candles. Those were times of relative austerity, but I remembered thoroughly enjoying our suitcase meals. The finest dining table could not have made life any more complete.

I could easily have responded quite differently to this situation. Had I thought that sitting on the floor and eating off a suitcase was a sign of deprivation, I would have felt embarrassed. If every time I sat down to dinner I ruminated about my lack of a proper table, most likely the food would not have been as palatable. This period of my life helped me understand that being happy does not depend on the number or quality of objects I own. Contentment comes from welcoming what is present, regardless of whether it fits our ideas about what will make us happy.

Santosha, the cultivation of contentment, is the second niyama. Contentment is deep acceptance of what is. Mindfulness practice, being present with and accepting each moment's unfolding phenomena, helps us to develop contentment on a fundamental level. As we practice mindfulness, we discover a natural sense of equanimity toward whatever is occurring in each moment. What arises is not negotiable; how we choose to respond to it is. In each moment, we have the opportunity to choose whether to meet our circumstances with acceptance or resistance. This choice sows the seeds of contentment or of suffering.

I have often found myself thinking that I will be happy only when things change—when I make more money, when I find the right relationship, when I can get a bigger house. Early in my asana practice, I speculated that I would be happier if I could touch my nose to the floor in seated forward bends or if I could accomplish the more "advanced" backbends. When these things came to pass, there was a moment of elation—it certainly felt great for my ego—followed by the realization that nothing had changed in my life as a result. I didn't even behave in a more enlightened way when I got stuck in traffic on the way home from class.

How many times have our desires been fulfilled in life? More times than we could remember. Where is the happiness of those fulfillments now? Quite often we do get what we hope for, but the happiness this brings is fleeting. Just like everything else in life, it is impermanent. Soon after we attain our latest goal, some new imagining becomes the panacea that will deliver us from the pain of wanting. Contentment doesn't depend on how many possessions or pleasurable experiences we have accumulated. It springs from our inner response to the full spectrum of experiences that we will all have in the span of our lives.

In 1989 I traveled to India to study at the Ramamani Iyengar Memorial Yoga Institute. Before I left, friends inundated me with stories of the terrible poverty, warning that I would be constantly depressed by the conditions there. What I found was certainly a way of life vastly different from mine. I can't imagine living in a corrugated metal shack without plumbing or electricity, as huge numbers of Pune's residents do. Any ideas I may have harbored about my own lack of wealth were put to rest when I remembered the reliable heat, water, and shelter of my tiny bungalow back in Utah.

But despite the overwhelming material poverty in India, I felt a dignity in the people there, a sense of self-worth that is not dependent on what they own, and this affected me as much as the poverty. I felt sad for the suffering that we in the wealthiest nation on the planet cause for ourselves by coveting huge mansions that we can't afford or cars that are newer or more expensive than our own. We also suffer when we consider ourselves worthy of admiration because of our comparative wealth. Or perhaps we have chosen a simple life and wear our lack of material wealth like a badge of honor, pronouncing ourselves morally superior to those who live extravagantly. These extremes cause us to feel isolated, and they obscure our intrinsic connectedness to others.

We all come into this world with different talents and abilities. Some of us are especially adept at creating wealth or are born into families that have accumulated wealth. Others of us are talented in disciplines that do not bring material abundance. All of us can appreciate and cultivate the particular talents we have and share them in a way that enlivens and enriches our lives. The world benefits from the interplay of all our unique abilities.

Contentment often feels unattainable because most of us believe we are inherently incomplete. The same feeling of lack that motivates greed and grasping obscures contentment. When you are truly present in this moment right now, is anything lacking? Mindfulness shows us that we are complete, albeit changing, beings. Our ideas about what will make us happy are all that stand in the way of being happy.

Practicing santosha not only brings greater satisfaction to our lives, it also supports the development of asteya (abundance) and aparigraha (letting go). When we understand that we are complete as we are, we cease grasping after what does not belong to us or holding fast to possessions, ideas, or lifestyles that no longer serve.

Being content with what is present does not mean that we must simply tolerate whatever situation we find ourselves in. But finding contentment even when our lives are difficult creates spaciousness around the difficulty. Mindfulness helps us find creative solutions and allows us to mine the jewels that inevitably appear when we navigate through challenging times.

Alistair Shearer's translation of Sutra II.42 says: "From contentment, unsurpassed happiness is gained." Contentment is the key that unlocks the possibility of enduring happiness. The deep satisfaction of santosha brings happiness that springs from within and is not shaken by the ever-changing landscapes of our lives.

Santosha in Your Asana Practice

Nothing creates greater dissatisfaction in asana practice than the thought that your practice should be something other than it is. You will receive the greatest benefit from practice when you stay present and appreciate where you are at this time. There is no guarantee that you will become enlightened when your head touches your knee in a forward bend or when you can achieve a full backbend! There is a possibility of greater freedom, though, if you relax your body and mind into your asanas just as they are.

Reflections

- Notice your response the next time you are forced to sit in a traffic jam, stand in line, or wait an inordinate amount of time to be served in a restaurant. Is your response adding to your suffering? What would it take to feel contented in this situation?

- How does cultivation of santosha relate to aparigraha and asteya? In what ways do these qualities feed each other?

- Reflect on all the things that have come to you in your life—all the wonderful experiences, material riches, close friendships, romantic relationships, and so on. Remember the happiness these things brought, and feel the emotions that arise as you remember. Is there something that you believe will make you happy now?

- Make a list of the things you appreciate in your life right now. Reflect on this list regularly, perhaps daily. Re-evaluate your list in three months. Note how your life has shifted. Make a new list, if appropriate, and check it again in three months.

- Sit and watch the breath. Watch carefully those moments when you feel connected to your breathing. In a moment of complete mindfulness, do you feel any desire?

Tapas: The Self-Generating Power of Discipline 15

MY FATHER was an amateur clarinetist. As far as I know, he had no aspirations to become a star performer. I don't recall him ever playing the sonatas he relentlessly practiced for any audience other than his family. The few times I remember him performing in public, it was as the bottom part of a woodwind trio, with my older sister and me. Nonetheless he practiced for an hour every evening without fail for many years. He devoted his Saturday mornings to teaching free half-hour clarinet lessons to interested high school students. He was an amateur in the literal sense: he played for pure love of his instrument.

As a budding oboist, my practice philosophy was quite different. In general, I slacked off most of the time and ramped up my practice when an important solo part was imminent and I was likely to embarrass myself with a shoddy performance. I mostly got away with this half-baked approach. I was willing to practice just enough to maintain my position as principal in the youth orchestra and felt lucky that I didn't have work very hard.

I marvel now at my father's unshakable discipline. There was no compelling reason for him to sit down every night and play the clarinet. He was not practicing to calm anxiety about the specter of some future performance. There were plenty of other things he could have done instead, and I suspect there were probably evenings when he didn't really feel like pulling out his instrument and plowing through his scales and arpeggios. But his practice time was nonnegotiable. Like all musicians, he did not start out proficient on his instrument. He invested years in woodshedding before playing for its own sake became enjoyable. Yet each tiny refinement in his tone and technique renewed his commitment to continue.

The discipline that compelled him to play clarinet each evening guided every aspect of my father's life. I have often thought that his haphazard, poverty-stricken, Depression-era upbringing inspired in him an strong desire to take control of his life. Unwavering commitment to everything he chose to accomplish was his way of keeping at bay the chaos of his past. As a result of his ardency, he became quite accomplished at an amazing array of endeavors in his relatively short lifetime.

Just as my father's discipline reached into other areas of his life, so did my lack of musical discipline mirror the rest of my life. In my schoolwork, I learned early on that I could procrastinate, rally at the last minute, and do just enough to make a respectable grade. I could not see the point of investing any more than the minimum amount of time and energy required to get by. While I loved playing music, drawing, and writing, whenever any of these things started to look like drudgery, I promptly backed away. It was not until I met Pujari that I understood the vitalizing power of discipline.

Tapas, which is often translated as discipline, is the third of the niyamas. The word has many translations, and the concept of tapas inspires a lot of interpretations, including austerity, discipline, simplicity, purification, and burning enthusiasm. I've come to understand tapas as a fabric interwoven with all these concepts, each one strengthening the others. I especially enjoy Kofi Busia's translation of Sutra II.43: "Inner ardour or determination perfects the body and the senses, and also destroys impurities." This translation expresses the fire-like quality of tapas that inspires practice as it consumes distractions.

I met Pujari and Abhilasha at a weekend workshop they taught in Salt Lake City in late 1985. At the time, I'd been practicing asana for almost four years. I'd become quite consistent in my daily routine; I rarely missed a day. However, despite my dedication to daily asana sessions, nothing much had changed in my practice ethic. I practiced only those poses that came easily. I had regained the flexibility of my youth but found myself sorely lacking in strength. I loved backbends, forward bends, and inversions, but standing poses were way too much work. Though my local teachers taught Iyengar-style asana, where standing poses were a weekly staple, I silently grumbled through these poses each week in order to get to the poses I liked.

Pujari's workshop changed my practice radically. Also a longtime student of B. K. S. Iyengar, Pujari began the first class of the weekend in typical Iyengar fashion, with an hour of nonstop standing poses. It was not his words—those I've long since forgotten—that caused the radical shift in me. Rather it was an undeniable, intense feeling of total commitment emanating from Pujari that inspired me to give no less than everything to my standing poses that night. I left the class energized and transformed.

For the next few years, I explored standing poses daily and with great enthusiasm. While the poses remained challenging, strength began to build, and the poses became an increasingly joyful experience. There were times when I felt like going back to my old way of practice, but it was no longer satisfying. I stayed committed to learning the art of standing poses and soon found that not only had my body become more grounded and strong, but I had become more resolute mentally and emotionally. I was standing on my own two feet in every way.

Having begun practice of the standing poses at such a rudimentary level, I had to concentrate on each technical baby step for months in order to gain the strength to move on to the next one. As a result, when I began teaching asana, I found the standing poses to be the ones I taught most thoroughly and proficiently. Starting at square one had allowed me to understand all the potential challenges along the way. This made me well equipped to anticipate my students' needs, much more so than in the poses that had come easily for me.

What changed during Pujari's workshop was the quality of attention and commitment that I brought to the practice. When I invested myself completely—mind, body, and heart—in the most difficult poses, there was no room for mental whining. The asana was the totality of my experience. Before, my practice had been pleasing but somewhat mechanical and rarely challenging. Attentiveness had catapulted my asana practice into unfamiliar and exciting territory. That mindfulness had created energy, energy generated enthusiasm, and enthusiasm inspired discipline. Daily standing practice brought new insights, which renewed my energy. I had discovered the self-generating power of tapas.

As my practice became enlivened through tapas, habits that no longer served my chosen direction began to fall away. I stopped using mind-altering drugs. In my college days, these substances had elevated my consciousness; now they left me feeling foggy and tired. Letting go of drugs simplified my life in many ways. I now had more resources to invest in my practice—a cleaner body–mind, which yielded more mental clarity and energy, as well as more money to attend workshops and classes. Gone was the ever-present, low-grade fear that I was doing something that could have grave consequences if I was caught. Seeing a police car on the street no longer produced an involuntary chill.

Habits of substance abuse do not fall away so easily in many cases, however. Some people have a stronger genetic predisposition toward addiction than others. In these cases, letting go of addiction can become your tapas practice. Asana and other mindfulness practices can be invaluable companions to other therapies.

My greatest challenge in practicing tapas has been learning to simplify my life. I've had to develop the discrimination to say no to things I want to do but can't comfortably fit into my schedule. For example, I'm often invited to play oboe in pick-up orchestras or as a guest in folk or chamber groups. These engagements always involve a series of rehearsals as well as performances. When I first began playing in Salt Lake, I always consented to these extra gigs. At times, I found myself rehearsing or performing every evening and spending hours each day practicing and making reeds, because my reeds wear out quickly when I'm rehearsing a lot. While I love playing music, and I consider it an important part of my life, when I over-commit to extra gigs, other practices—including asana, meditation, and writing—diminish drastically.

In recent years, I've learned to quell my compulsion to consent to every engagement that comes along. I began by saying no to the ones that I knew would not be interesting musically. What has been more challenging is turning down engagements that I know would be fun and inspiring. I only consent to play extra concerts now when I can do so without limiting other important practices. I also no longer accept extra gigs at the expense of my downtime.

Tapas then is a discipline of balancing our lives so that we invest our resources wisely. Much of practicing tapas is developing the art of discernment, determining which of our daily commitments support the general direction of our evolutionary track and which ones do not. As with the other yamas and niyamas, moderation supports healthy practice. Practicing tapas should not turn us into automatons for yoga. Being monomaniacal about practice is not healthy. Rather, we learn to live with our most compelling priorities in mind, even as we allow ourselves the freedom to explore occasional diversions.

Pujari suggests that asana and meditation practitioners commit to doing five minutes each day. This amount of practice time is available to virtually everyone. In the heat of beginner's zeal, practitioners often vow to practice an hour or more each day. Very quickly this can become an all-or-nothing proposition. When we find this goal unattainable, we often quit practicing altogether and judge ourselves harshly for what we perceive to be our failure. Five minutes a day is consistently doable, and it often grows into a longer practice when time is available. Discipline can be developed, even for the most scattered of us, but it must evolve with wisdom and patience.

I've found tapas to be a meld of discipline, simplicity, mindfulness, and enthusiasm. With discipline, we steadily feed our aspirations. As our practice grows, extraneous, unsupportive distractions fall away. Our lives become simpler. Simplicity brings our paths into sharper focus, which allows us to invest our consciousness more mindfully to our tasks. Mindfulness generates insight, energy, and enthusiasm, which renew our resolve to practice.

Although it is often helpful to adhere to a practice schedule, the structure and time allotment of your practice matters much less than the presence you bring to it. Mindfulness creates the energy and interest needed to sustain consistent practice. It also helps you identify distractions that deplete your time and energy. Invest yourself totally in all your daily practices, from asana to washing dishes. Watch your relationship to yourself evolve.

Tapas in Your Asana Practice

Commit to daily asana practice. If you are very busy, resolve to practice for an amount of time that you know you can fit into your schedule. Even five minutes a day is beneficial. Make this time sacrosanct; avoid letting your practice time be overshadowed by other things. Of course, you may practice longer if time permits. If you want to build tapas, it is more beneficial to practice daily for short periods than it is to practice once a week for two hours. Consistency builds commitment. Even if your practice is only five minutes long, invest all your energy into it.

Practice a new pose each week. It is easy to fall into a rut while practicing. This can make practice less interesting. Mix a few less familiar poses into your routine.

Reflections

- Schedule your asana and meditation practice for a time when you are least likely to be disturbed by family, friends, or the phone. Better yet, turn the phone ringer off during your practice.

- Make an inventory of your daily commitments. Which are the most important to you? Consider what responsibilities you might give up or spend less time on. Where can you reinvest this energy that will best serve your deepest aspirations?

- Make room in your life for downtime. Find a few minutes each day to do nothing. Does this practice require more or less discipline than the previous two?

- How are aparigraha, saucha, and santosha related to tapas? Reflect on how these practices can strengthen each other in your life.

Svadhyaya: 16
Refining Wisdom

A FEW YEARS into my asana practice, I bought B. K. S. Iyengar's book *Light on the Yoga Sutras of Patanjali*. A teaching colleague had begun sutra study, and I felt duty-bound to keep up. This phase of my early yoga career lasted about one hour. Though my intellect understood many of the sutras as I read them, once I'd read them they completely slipped out of my mind. Their impact was much less than I had hoped. I decided that I really didn't need to read the sutras in order to understand yoga. I would simply practice. Later I would discover this decision to be an expression of accidental wisdom.

In the ensuing years, I practiced asana with diligence, and in 1988 I sat my first vipassana retreat. In addition to endless hours of sitting and walking, twice each day of the retreat we listened to taped discourses by wise and insightful teachers like Joseph Goldstein, Sharon Salzberg, Steven Armstrong, and Michele McDonald. These talks not only brought relief from having to witness the irritating parade of garbage rambling on and on in my mind, but they helped clarify and even pacify some of my reactions to it. These teachers related personal experiences not so different from my own and helped me understand the universality of the experience of an untrained mind. From the discourses, I learned about the underlying causes of much of my mental discomfort and learned ways to create the space to work with them. When I returned home I immediately got a catalog from Dharma Seed Tape Library and ordered a dozen tapes. I have listened to these talks (and many others purchased over the years) again and again. I have continued to glean new bits of wisdom from them as my own meditative understanding has deepened.

A few years ago, I received an e-mail advertisement from a yoga studio that touted yoga as the "latest fitness craze" and offered classes that were free of the "spiritual baggage." Spiritual baggage! Suddenly I found myself feeling protective of the larger yoga tradition, even though I had not attempted to read the sutras in years. I went to a couple of local bookstores and came home with ten more translations. I cleared a space for them on my bookshelf, and there they remained, unopened, until a fortuitous meeting with an old acquaintance a month later.

One crisp summer Sunday afternoon, I was returning from a hike up Mt. Aire, a peak in the Wasatch Mountain range on Salt Lake City's eastern border. As I made my way down the steep trail, I glimpsed what I thought was a familiar face. Simultaneously the face turned to look at me. It was Lorie, a friend I'd worked with for several years at a natural foods store in the late 1980s. Lorie's mother, Margaret Hahn, is a longtime yoga teacher in Omaha, and as a child Lorie had accompanied her mother on several excursions to Iyengar's institute in Pune. When I worked with her at the store, she did not practice. Now, it turned out, she had returned to yoga and was interested in studying the sutras. We resolved to study together and have met monthly ever since.

As we began reading, I was interested to discover that the Yoga Sutras, while organized somewhat differently, are almost identical to the Buddhist philosophy I'd been reading for so many years. Moreover, after years of practice, many of the concepts presented by the sutras were already anchored in my experience. Unlike my first abortive attempt at sutra study years before, now the sutras commented upon and clarified my understanding. I've found the meetings with Lorie and the study in between to be invaluable, and the wisdom of the sutras has appeared in my teaching in unexpected ways.

The fourth niyama, svadhyaya, is commonly translated as either "self-study" or "study of spiritual texts." In my experience, self-study and the study of spiritual literature are interwoven. Without self-study, yogic and Buddhist philosophy (or that of any other spiritual system), while certainly comprehensible at the level of intellect, is not particularly relatable to one's life experience. Self-study, without taking advantage of the wisdom of those who have passed before, can be confusing and can sometimes get bogged down in self-obsession. Texts such as the Yoga Sutras point to the universality of our experience and connect us with a wider understanding of it.

My favorite translation of Sutra II.44 is from T. K. V. Desikachar: "Study, when it is developed to the highest degree, brings one close to higher forces that promote understanding of the most complex." This translation does not limit svadhyaya to a specific type of study but points to the power of the two wings of study to move us closer to understanding those concepts he calls "the most complex," those not readily accessible to the intellect alone.

Like any other practice, continued study, through the avenues of mindfulness and the wisdom of our teachers, weaves understanding into the fabric of our being. Moreover each reading of the sutras, like each listening of my beloved dharma tapes, yields new discoveries as my self-understanding deepens.

Before I left for a three-week vipassana retreat in 2003, I read the introduction to Alistair Shearer's sutra translation, *The Yoga Sutras of Patanjali*. When I returned from retreat, I reread the introduction. This time I highlighted paragraphs on almost every page and tagged more than thirty pages with sticky notes. In just three weeks of intense mindfulness practice, my relationship to the text transformed. I saw it with new eyes. I look forward to future readings of the introduction and the sutras I've already studied and to discovering the jewels still lying in wait.

Svadhyaya in Your Asana Practice

The most meaningful way to discover the benefits of asana is to experience them directly, by using your own body as a laboratory for exploration. My favorite way to teach myself and my students to understand the effects of asana on their physical, mental, and emotional well-being is to begin practice in a neutral pose. This could be Sukkhasana (Cross-Legged Sitting Pose), Tadasana (Mountain Pose), or Savasana (Relaxation Pose)

As you sit, stand, or lie in one of these poses, feel how your b to gravity, whether your weight is evenly distributed over yo and back body. Notice the quality of your energy. Is it agit quick or sluggish, moving up or moving down? Perform an asana, and then come back to your neutral position. Assess your energy again. Has anything changed? Continue practicing in this way, returning to neutral after each pose. Watch the evolution of your physical, mental, and emotional energies.

Reflections

- If you feel moved to study the Yoga Sutras or to read about meditation, keep in mind that the wisdom that underlies these texts evolves with you. Your own internal explorations in practice provide the essential tools for integrating yogic wisdom into your being.

- Find a study partner, or sponsor a study group. Hearing other people's interpretations of the sutras fleshes out your understanding. Set a date each month to meet and discuss what you've learned.

- Choose several translations to study. The differences in interpretation can be surprising. Each shows us a different angle to consider. Lorie and I base our study on Alistair Shearer's translation and complement it with other translations. I have listed my favorite translations in Resources.

- The sutras are divided into sections of as few as two or three up to a half dozen aphorisms. Study one section each month.

- Lorie writes each month's sutras on a card and laminates it so she can take it with her wherever she goes. This is a great way to keep the sutras in mind as you move through your day.

- From time to time, revisit sutras you've already read. Note whether or how your understanding has changed.

Ishvarapranidhana: 17
Surrendering to Grace

WHEN I FIRST BEGAN teaching asana, I spent the hour before each class writing down exactly what I wanted to present. To the left of each asana on the list I wrote the approximate amount of time it would take, and to the right I listed technical details I did not want to forget. While I never repeated a previous class, I kept all my class plans in a notebook for future reference.

Structuring my classes helped me clarify my intentions for the class and create an arc that I hoped would leave students feeling balanced. I followed my outlines meticulously. After class I evaluated what I felt had worked and what hadn't and marked the page accordingly. I learned a lot about pacing and class flow this way.

My first vipassana retreat happened about a year and a half after I began teaching. When I returned from retreat, I came to class prepared with an outline I felt was especially creative and inspired. But when I entered the classroom, I sensed that what I had planned was not really what the class needed at that time. As much as I wanted to hew to my outline, my heart would not allow it. After a moment of trepidation, I took what felt like a giant leap into no-man's-land. I closed my notebook and began teaching spontaneously. Throughout the class, I felt insecure, groundless, not knowing what would come next, but each pose flowed into the next seamlessly. Sentences leapt out of my mouth, words and concepts I'd never before considered. I was clearly not in charge of this class. I felt I was simply a vessel through which yoga was expressing itself. Teaching a class without a safety net invigorated me in a way that my planned classes never had.

Convinced this was a fluke, two days later I returned to my notebook to outline my next class. But as I began that day's class, I again realized that my preplanned agenda was not what the students needed. I surrendered control and allowed the class to flow through me. Again I felt completely insecure, but the class came to life in its own way. As two days previously, the things I said surprised me, and as much as I wanted to remember them for future use, by the end of class I could not retrieve them. It took another six months for me to trust enough to skip preparing outlines, even though I never again used them for an ongoing weekly class. (I do still plan subjects for workshops and retreats, but I'm always open to letting these evolve spontaneously if need be.)

In giving up the security of my outline, I was no longer limited by its parameters. I felt as if I was stepping into the current of a great river of universal wisdom. I realized that this tributary was constantly present, that it had cascaded through all of time. No matter how hard I had worked to find the mysterious flow that I had experienced in some of the workshops with other teachers, and regardless of the level of perfection of my yogic technique, in the end all I had to do was relax, let go, and simply step into it. It had never been separate from me.

Ishvarapranidhana, the fifth niyama, is often translated as "surrender or devotion to God." This translation, with its monotheistic implications, has required a lot of contemplation for me. I've never connected with the idea of an ever-present, all-knowing god. For me, it has been those times in my life when I felt fully present but no longer in charge—in the spontaneous yoga classes as well as while playing music, walking in the desert, gardening, sitting in meditation, even dancing at Grateful Dead concerts—that I have felt connected with a sense of wisdom greater than my own. Swami Venkatesananda offers a translation that best reflects my understanding of ishvarapranidhana. His sutra translation reads: "Perfection in self-awareness instantly follows total, dynamic and intelligent surrender of the individual ego-sense (in the sense of the realization of its unreal nature) or the merging of it in the indwelling omnipresence (in the sense of the direct realization of the falsity of the 'me,' the ego-sense, and therefore the sole reality of the indwelling omnipresence)."

It took several readings at different times for me to digest this translation, and I imagine I'll read it many more times before I fully understand it. For now, here's what I think: The realization of the unreal nature of the ego-sense is the recognition that my belief in the reality of myself as an individual personality is illusory. When I surrender this belief in a defined ego-self, and therefore surrender that ego-self's need to be in control, that individual self dissolves into the "indwelling omnipresence," the settled mind, or the infinite river of wisdom.

This surrender happens when we invest our total presence into whatever we are doing. So again, we return to mindfulness. It is mindfulness that allows us to experience our lives directly, without the intervening presence of the ego and its conditioned judgments.

Practicing surrendering to grace does not necessarily mean that we should leap blindly into situations we know nothing about. I speculate that ishvarapranidhana is listed as the last of the niyamas because it must be grounded in our practice of the yamas and the other niyamas. Without the foundation of saucha, santosha, tapas, and svadhyaya, surrender might lead to chaos. I could not have effectively taught without a class plan had I not trained for so many years before. It was the integration of my committed asana practice and the many hours spent on producing and studying my outlines that allowed me to improvise without leading the class into confusion and entropy. The previous niyamas teach us to set intentions and invest energy and discipline into carrying them out. The yamas and niyamas provide the lifejacket that allows us to swim in the flow of the river without being swept under.

Practicing ishvarapranidhana requires that we give up our need to control. Control is an illusion. The evidence is everywhere. Sit and watch your mind for one minute. Are you inviting the thoughts and sensations you feel? Can you control the sensations and thoughts that enter your mind? Consider your own body. Aging happens despite all our efforts to stifle it. I did not will my hair to go gray, my joints to creak when I get out of bed in the morning, or my skin to become drier by the year. These things simply happened, in blatant opposition to my wishes.

Even the things I endeavor to accomplish are not under my control. All I can do is take steps toward my dreams and then surrender to the outcome. Instead of suffering disappointment when my expectations are not perfectly fulfilled, I can appreciate the often surprising results—results that are often much more rewarding than what I could have imagined. When I give up control, I may at times fall, but I've learned that magic does not occur within my ego's walled-in compound. Ishvarapranidhana asks us to trust in what we cannot see or know. When we practice surrender, we dwell in grace.

Ishvarapranidhana in Your Asana Practice

During asana practice, we can be fully present with the direct experience of each pose, with all the sensations that occur, beginning with our intention to practice a particular pose. Here's how it works: Move slowly enough to feel the tiny, incremental movements that make up your transition into the formal pose. Stay in the pose long enough to feel how the body's relationship to it evolves. How does your body movement relate to your breath movement? What is the qualitative difference in your experience between pushing your body toward a preconceived goal (under the direction of the executive ego) and surrendering continually to the reality of the pose as it is right now? Stay present for the transitional movements as you come out of the pose. Then sit, stand, or lie in a neutral position for a few breaths afterward to note how the pose has changed you.

Reflections

- If you have cultivated a garden, raised a child, or shared a household with animal companions, reflect on the ways in which they have and have not conformed to your expectations. How can you balance your desire to steer their lives in a skillful direction with the practice of ishvarapranidhana?

- Do something you've never done before. Attend a lecture or documentary on a subject you know nothing about, or attend a concert of unfamiliar music. Do something radical, like signing up for a dance class (if you've never danced) or a rock-climbing workshop. Travel somewhere you would never have considered going. Even driving home from work via a different route can help defuse the fear of the unfamiliar. Doing something outside your comfortable routine helps develop the courage to surrender to the unknown.

The Third Limb
Asana: Abiding in Ease

18

ASANA. Perhaps it should be called *ahhhsana*, for its tendency to produce sighs of pleasure. No matter what we call it, the profound, pleasing, transcendent, or transformative sensations that often accompany asana practice are probably the primary reason you were interested enough in the eight limbs of yoga to pick up this book. In Western culture, asana is the gateway to all the other practices that make up the eight limbs. We begin our exploration in the physical realm and soon find that, as the body goes, so goes the mind.

In two decades of teaching, I've observed that the most common motivators that bring people to asana classes are a need to alleviate back pain, a wish to gain strength and flexibility, and a desire to counter the effects of stress, such as insomnia, high blood pressure, and general edginess. Practicing asana has the potential to bring about all these benefits. Over many years of practice, I've witnessed powerful and unexpected healing, stabilization, and grace developing in my own body and in those of students and colleagues. What yogis often do not realize until they've practiced for many years is that asana can yield benefits on a grand scope, not just in the moment of practice but as we move through our lives.

At this writing, a Google search on the benefits of yoga yields more than 10,200,000 pages. While I admit I perused only a small number of them, none of the pages I read listed the primary benefit outlined by the Yoga Sutras, a benefit I find to be extraordinary. Alistair Shearer's translation of Sutra II.48, the third of the three sutras devoted to the third limb (asana), explains that once asana is mastered "we are no longer upset by the play of opposites."

During one long and confusing day, which happened to be my birthday, I experienced this benefit of practice in a powerful way. The day was sunny and seventy degrees. Thoughtful friends and relatives treated me to phone calls and surprise visits. I felt showered with love and good wishes throughout the day. With each greeting, I felt thankful for the gift of the many wonderful friendships in my life.

Despite the crystalline skies and perfect spring temperature, I spent most of the day hiding indoors. My next-door neighbor, who suffers from schizoaffective disorder and had not been medicated in many years, was on a rampage. I could not walk outside without meeting with an unpleasant encounter. He threw snails at me—snails he claimed belonged to me and were invading his yard. He shouted unrepeatable epithets. He charged after my partner, Phillip, as he walked down the street. The ordeal finally ended after our third call to police. Upon returning home after a lovely meal at one of my favorite restaurants, we found my neighbor standing at my property line, shirtless in the dark, swinging a golf club over his head and swearing at us. The police witnessed this and arrested him for aggravated assault.

After a day of ricocheting from one extreme to the other—from gratitude to fear and back many times over—I felt completely spent. For much of the day, my nervous system was on edge, in fight-or-flight mode. By my last encounter with the police, my body was trembling uncontrollably. Still, as I talked with the police, I was able to speak calmly, precisely, and rationally. When I sat down to meditate that night, I was present with the physical, mental, and emotional ravages the day had wrought. At the same time, the awareness that was present with the state of my frazzled nervous system was not shaken. Awareness, the settled mind, provided refuge from the chaos in my body–mind. I felt enormous gratitude for my asana and meditation practices and the ballast they had provided me while traversing such turbulent waters.

Through the vehicle of the physical practice, asana balances the nervous system, creating a quiet environment into which the mind can settle. I once heard Judith Hanson Lasater say, "If you want to change your mind, change your body." The mind and body are inextricably woven together. What you do to the body cannot help but affect the mind. When the body is agitated, it is much more difficult for the mind to settle. When the body is calm, the mind is more likely to relax.

As a culture, we spend much of our time in the sympathetic nervous system, the fight-or-flight side of our autonomic nervous system. We race from one appointment to the next. We live in our cars, constantly aware that one unconscious move by us or another driver could cause serious injury or death. We are continually on edge. The sympathetic nervous system serves a very important function. It dilates our pupils and speeds our respiration and heartbeat. It shunts most of our blood away from our extremities and vital organs and into the big muscles of the body, the muscles we need to run from predators. (This is why food is difficult to digest when we are under stress.) The sympathetic nervous system makes it possible for us to avoid imminent peril. However, when we live almost continuously in our sympathetic nervous system, we become depleted and vulnerable to stress-related disease.

In a perfect world, we would live most of the time in the parasympathetic side, the "rest and digest" side of the nervous system. In parasympathetic mode, our heart beats more slowly and steadily, our breathing is relaxed, and our blood circulates through our internal organs to support our vital functions. There we replenish and regenerate the body–mind.

Continued asana practice changes the body–mind at a fundamental level. Over time, the practice of relaxing the body, marrying its movements with deep, full breathing, changes the nervous system, making us more resilient. Our minds are better able to stay calm, no matter what difficulties might be present. The slow, mindful movements of asana practice suppress the sympathetic nervous system and allow us to dwell in the parasympathetic nervous system.

Practicing asana also gives us greater access to the awareness that underlies the movements of our minds. This neutral, unchanging awareness is what allowed me to stay calm throughout the extremes that occurred on my birthday. It was absolutely appropriate for my body to respond by flipping into fight-or-flight mode throughout the day. The danger was real. But instead of losing my mental and emotional grip, I was able to access a fundamental stillness and still appreciate the times of the day that were indeed quite lovely.

We all experience the play of opposites in our lives: pleasure and pain, gain and loss, praise and blame, and fame and disrepute. Sometimes, as on my birthday, we can swing between them many times, even in the span of a single day. Experiencing these opposites is part of being human. This is the very reason the Buddha claimed human birth to be such a precious opportunity for evolution. Living as a human being gives us ample opportunity to experience the pain that can lead to deeper inquiry, tempered with enough pleasure to keep us from giving up. Human birth provides the perfect balance of the factors for moving toward enlightenment.

While practicing the yamas and niyamas can help us avert potential conflict, the fact is that most of what happens in our lives is out of our control. Balancing our responses to life's vicissitudes is far more crucial to our happiness than the unlikely possibility that we could somehow control the events in our lives so that we experience only happy ones.

How can a physical practice help us to remain undisturbed by the play of opposites in our lives? Equanimity comes not from performing increasingly impressive feats on the mat. It comes from how we approach the poses we practice, regardless of whether our practice is simple or complicated.

The first asana-based sutra tells us how we can approach practice in a way that cultivates equanimity. Shearer's translation of Sutra II.46 is: "The physical posture should be steady and comfortable." Other translations use the phrases "firm and pleasant," "alertness and relaxation," "steady and easy" and "firm and soft," all of which can be interpreted as pairs of opposing qualities. If we practice with the intention to maintain a balance of steadiness and comfort or firmness and softness, we cultivate the ability to remain centered while dancing between opposites.

As I understand this sutra, the aspect of a practitioner that must be firm or steady is his or her resolve to stay in an asana even when difficulty arises. In order to lengthen a muscle in the long term, we must hold a position for a minimum of thirty seconds. In each bundle of muscle cells is a sensory nerve called the muscle spindle sensory nerve. Its function is to sense when a muscle is being stretched beyond its capacity. When the muscle spindle nerve senses danger, it sends a message to the spinal cord, which in turn sends a message through the muscle's motor neurons to protect the muscle by shortening it. After thirty seconds, the muscle spindle nerve habituates to its new length and no longer sends a message of distress to the spinal cord. This allows the muscle to maintain its length.

If we never stay in a pose long enough to inquire into and make peace with the discomfort that can arise, how can we expect to find the equanimity to remain undisturbed by the difficulties in our lives? We hold each pose long enough to get to know the nature of our discomfort. This can yield valuable insights. The first is that everything changes. As we relax into a pose, the sensations we feel shift. They move; they lighten or intensify; new sensations arise. Observing the transitory nature of body sensation teaches us to look beneath the surface appearance of things. We learn by experience that no matter how pleasant or unpleasant our present situation is, it will not continue as it is. This understanding can only happen when we commit to spending some time in each pose.

Sometimes asana practice evokes uncomfortable emotions. For the first seven years of my practice, I felt extreme anxiety when I practiced Paschimottanasana (Seated Forward Bend). The fear was primal; I felt suffocated in the pose. Every time I practiced I would take myself just to the edge of the fear and then come out, a process that usually lasted considerably less than thirty seconds. One day, I set a firm resolve to stay no matter what happened. The fear turned to intense panic, but I remained steady in my resolve and continued to soften my body and mind around the anxiety. After several minutes, the fear dissolved and has never returned.

In telling this story, I'm not recommending that you jump right into eradicating all difficult emotional responses from your practice immediately. Sometimes it is wise simply to note that certain poses evoke certain emotions. You can test these waters gently, increasing your endurance by a few seconds with each practice. Or there may be days, weeks, or years when you don't practice an emotionally evocative pose at all.

Mindfulness of your present energy level is essential here. Do you have the energy to face a difficult emotion, or is it best to note it and back away? This creates a perfect opportunity to practice right effort. While I have no way of proving this, I'm certain that I could not have moved into my fear in Paschimottanasana any sooner than I did. After seven years of practice, I had developed enough self-awareness to know that I was ready at that time and not a moment sooner.

When I first began practicing yoga in the Iyengar tradition, I generally resented all the emphasis on alignment. I preferred the "flow and glow" school. I didn't want to bother with setting up all those pesky props. The constant chatter about minute details irritated me. I didn't care if my pose was perfect. I just wanted to feel good.

Yet for some reason I stayed with the method. Gradually I began to realize that attention to alignment is not about creating a perfect pose, whatever that is. It is, on the most superficial level, about creating a condition that allows the body to move into positions outside its normal parameters without causing injury. Awareness of alignment also allowed me to discover the areas of my body that were chronically out of alignment, so I could begin to unwind habits that might cause injury in the future. Finally, alignment awareness created a more even flow of the subtle energies throughout the body, which in turn brought my body–mind into a profound state of balance during and after practice. Alignment is about practicing with integrity.

Over years of practice, I've developed a method for balancing steadiness with comfort in my asana practice. Each asana begins with the first inkling of intention to perform it. This is where I begin applying mindfulness. Because the process of moving into an asana is just as important as the formal position itself, I stay present with the transition into the pose, adjusting my body as I go, to allow for optimum alignment integrity. Then I stop for a few breaths in a manifestation of the asana that is comfortable for me. Here I assess where my body is today, because no matter how many times in my life I may have placed my body in this particular form, whether it's Adho Mukha Svanasana (Downward-Facing Dog Pose), Utthita Trikonasana (Extended Triangle Pose), or another of my staples, I have never before performed this pose in this moment. A beginner's mind is invaluable.

Then, if it feels appropriate, I begin to move slowly and attentively toward my edge, always maintaining alignment integrity. When I reach the point where I feel challenged but—and this is crucial—where my breathing is still easy and full, I relax. As I inhale, new space opens in my body; as I exhale, I relax into that space. Perhaps my edge shifts, perhaps it doesn't. Either way, I breathe and relax into the present reality of the asana.

In this way, I am moving cooperatively with my body, not forcing it beyond its present capacity. This allows my nervous system to remain calm. And most important, I learn how to soften into the edge of what I'm willing to be with. This trains me to maintain equanimity no matter what challenges I might face in my life. When I'm ready to release the asana, I make a mindful transition toward a neutral pose, such as standing, sitting, or lying. Here I allow myself to feel the effects of the asana.

Deepening into an asana may or may not mean that your body moves more fully into the formal pose. Rather, deepening is about continually relaxing into the asana as it is. As you deepen into an asana, you are no longer doing it; you become the asana. This state of being the asana is described in the next sutra.

Sutra II.47 defines mastery of asana, saying (according to Shearer's translation): "[Asanas] are mastered when all effort is relaxed and the mind is absorbed in the Infinite." An asana is realized when we have reached a level of relaxation that allows us to accept our pose as complete in each moment, regardless of whether it bears any resemblance to our idealized concepts of what it should be. When we understand that the asana is whole as it is, we cease to apply effort. Continual relaxation into the present reality of a pose allows our mind to settle into silence.

Mastery then has nothing to do with physical prowess. Whether we ever perform a thirty-minute Salamba Sirsasana (Headstand), a straight-armed Urdhva Dhanurasana (Upward-Facing Bow Pose), or a perfect Salabhasana (Locust Pose) is irrelevant. Mastery depends on the quality of attention, and the quality of intention, we bring to practice. Here we can draw upon ahimsa (so we respect our body's limits and, through our desire not to harm, stay within them) and santosha (so we can be content with our practice as it is).

Judith Hanson Lasater translates Sutra II.46 as "Abiding in ease is asana." To me, this translation sums up the purpose of asana practice—to live in a state of ease, no matter what is happening in our lives. In this way, we can remain fully open to the play of opposites we all endure. Asana practice is our training ground. It balances our nervous system, creating a calm physical environment for our minds, and it teaches us how to relax into life's challenges. Pain is unavoidable; struggle is always of our own making. We struggle when we fight against what is present. Asana teaches us how to effect change by relaxing into each situation, so that we can respond to our lives in fresh, creative, and intelligent ways.

Asana in Your Asana Practice

In a recent workshop with Judith Hanson Lasater, each asana class began and ended with the chanting of Sutra II.46 in Sanskrit: "shtira sukkham asanam." I like this practice because it clarifies an intention to practice asana in a way that creates physical, mental, and emotional equilibrium.

As you chant vocally or repeat the sutra silently, set an intention to practice keeping Sutra II.46 in mind. As you practice each asana, notice if the body and mind are steady and comfortable (or firm and soft, steady and easy, alert and relaxed—whichever words suit you). Notice how being steady and comfortable expresses itself in each pose.

For example, in standing poses, it is likely to help if the legs are steady so that the upper body can be comfortable. Is there struggle anywhere in the body or mind? Perhaps the struggle is due to giving primacy to accomplishment of the pose rather than to ease. Or maybe the body is struggling because the parts of the body that form the foundation of the pose—those parts that are in contact with the ground—are not truly supporting you.

In what parts of the body are you struggling needlessly? I often see students clenching their jaws or hunching their shoulders while practicing challenging poses. It's likely that these are habitual responses to stress that also manifest in their daily lives. It is not helpful to imprint these patterns into your asana practice. Rather, asana practice offers the opportunity to identify the areas you habitually tighten and to choose to let them relax.

Reflections

- Choose and practice a pose that you find easy and pleasurable and one that you find challenging or unpleasant. Note your responses to each. Are you attached to the pleasurable pose? Do you dislike the less pleasant one? Relax into both poses, and relax into your responses to them. Include both poses in your practice for a month. Note at the end of the month if your relationship with them has changed. Decide whether you want to continue working with these two poses or move on to new ones.

■ Commit to steadiness in your relationship with your practice. Practice every day for a month, committing to an amount of time that fits your schedule. If five minutes a day is all you can commit to, enjoy those five minutes to the fullest. After a month, take a day or two off. What do you notice when you return to practice? What do you notice in your life off the mat?

■ Practice with books that inspire you and remind you of alignment concepts. In the Resources section, I've listed a few of the books I find useful. Work with a single book for a period of time, so that you give yourself the opportunity to integrate its viewpoints and information. There are many good books available about asana. The ones I've included are just the ones I'm most familiar with. Remember, working with an experienced teacher who can give you feedback on your alignment is far more effective than practicing solely with books or videos.

■ If you are a long-term practitioner, reflect every six months or so how your practice has changed over time. How has your primary intention for practice shifted? Are there poses you used to love that no longer fit? Are there poses you once found tedious or difficult that have become allies? Write down your observations and revisit them periodically.

The Fourth Limb
Pranayama: Expanding Life Force

19

THE HOUSE where I grew up stood at the edge of a small woods. My sisters and I spent most of our playtime outside, creating imaginary worlds among the trees. Even now, I remember the landmarks along what seemed like an endless trail—a huge sycamore tree with a rope swing suspended from a high branch, a grove of trees tangled together with vines, a slight rise in the path that signaled the nearness of one of the woods' great centerpieces, the hole camp. This was a hole in the ground that neighborhood kids had partly covered with logs, making an underground shelter. The hole camp assumed many identities over the years, from secret hideout to gilded mansion, depending on what our fantasies required. Reflecting on the myriad exotic identities of this rather crude hole in the ground, it is evident that being in the vastness of the outdoors opened our creative minds.

I still love being outside. A hike in the mountains renews me. Here in Utah, the rarefied mountain air seems to buzz. When I walk in the mountains, my senses sharpen. My vision becomes vivid; even the smallest pebbles and most delicate wildflower petals emerge into sharp—almost surreal—focus. Bird song, rustling leaves, the buzz of horseflies, and the scrambling of prairie rodents create a tranquil and surprising symphony.

Being in nature enlivens because it places us in the midst of the essential force that animates all living things. Yogis call this force *prana*. Prana exists everywhere, from the stones of the earth to the fiery stars, and in all flora and fauna. It permeates the air. It is the universal energy. In his book *The Complete Illustrated Book of Yoga*, Swami Vishnu-devananda explains,

"Prana is in all forms of matter and yet it is not matter. It is the energy or force that animates matter."

We imbibe this energy through the food and water we consume and the air we breathe. However, as Vishnu-devananda points out, food, water, and air in themselves are not prana; they are simply the vehicles through which we draw in this life force and distribute it throughout all our cells. He writes, "Prana is in the air, but it is not the oxygen, nor any of its chemical constituents. It is in food, water, and in the sunlight, yet it is not vitamin, heat, or light-rays. Food, water, air, etc., are only the media through which the prana is carried."

We spend our prana when we move, speak, and think, in the mundane acts that make up our daily lives. We must travel from place to place, commuting to work, shopping for food, tending the garden, and keeping our indoor space clean and clear. Maintaining silence in our daily lives is not practical. Communicating with our friends, family, and coworkers is not only necessary, but it can be a great pleasure. And the thinking mind is an essential tool in organizing our lives. Thought-based activities, such as reading and writing, stimulate our minds in infinitely positive ways. Engaging in all these things requires that we spend our prana.

According to Swami Vishnu-devananda, practicing pranayama is the most efficient way to replenish our essential life force. Often translated as "breath control," pranayama in Alistair Shearer's translation implies expansion rather than restraint. The Sanskrit word for life force is *prana*. When combined with the word *yama*, which we already know is associated with control or restraint of our behavior, control of the life force is implied. But Shearer suggests that *prana* is combined with the word *ayama*, which means to expand or increase. According to this interpretation, *pranayama* literally means the expansion of our vital life energy. Normal breathing keeps us alive but does not increase our prana. According to the sutras, it is through the breathing practices developed by yogis over millennia that we extend our life energy.

Sutra II.49 says (according to Shearer): "Next [after asana] come the breathing exercises, which suspend the flow of breath and increase the life energy." Sutra II.50 further explains: "The life energy is increased by regulation of the out-breath, the in-breath, or the breath in mid-flow. Depending upon the volume, and the length and frequency of holding, the breathing becomes slow and refined."

The sutras are deliberately vague here, addressing theory rather than the practice of pranayama, because these practices are best learned from a knowledgeable teacher. In more than two decades of practice, I've learned pranayama techniques from an array of teachers, all of whom teach from their own highly individual experiences, and I've heard a lot of conflicting information from one teacher to the next. I'm sure that all the techniques are helpful for some people in some situations, but as in every practice, we must consider what we bring to pranayama before launching headlong into this powerful practice.

Ultimately the most fruitful route for me has been to explore each teacher's advice and feel its effects in my own body–mind over time. Then I can decide in an informed way which practices are appropriate for me at a given stage. I've found that techniques are not especially helpful, however, if our everyday, underlying breathing pattern is inefficient or unhealthy.

When I studied with the Iyengars in Pune in 1989, we practiced asana for three hours each morning and pranayama for up to two hours each afternoon. Despite many hours of pranayama practice, I accomplished exactly one deep, satisfying inhalation during the three weeks of the intensive. Needless to say, the pranayama practice felt very frustrating to me. While my commitment to asana grew by leaps and bounds as a result of my India experience, I abruptly abandoned pranayama practice as soon as I left Pune.

I did not realize then that in practicing pranayama I was attempting to layer breathing techniques onto an essentially inefficient habitual breathing pattern. All my life I'd been a chest breather, which is not only inefficient but is unhealthy as well. Instead of allowing my abdomen to expand on the inhale and deflate on the exhale, I pulled in my belly on the inhale, simultaneously heaving open my chest, and on the exhale I returned my belly to a tentative state of relaxation while collapsing my chest. While I can't pinpoint exactly what made me deviate from natural abdominal breathing, I suspect it was a fear of appearing to have a belly that caused me to want to keep my abdominal muscles in almost continuous contraction.

This type of breathing is inefficient because it employs the small, secondary respiratory located in the neck and shoulders to do the work of the much larger and stronger primary respiratory muscles—the diaphragm, the abdominals, and the intercostals (the muscles between the ribs). In healthy abdominal breathing, the primary respiratory muscles support normal respiration, while the secondary muscles help us inhale extra air when we become winded from aerobic activity. The secondary muscles also take over respiratory duties while we're in deep sleep, when the body needs less oxygen. Chest breathing restricts the motion of the primary respiratory muscles, making deep, satisfying breathing virtually impossible.

When a newborn baby breathes, her entire body expands and contracts as she inhales and exhales, distributing life-giving prana throughout. This constant oscillation is the basic motion that underlies all other movements. Vishnu-devananda calls the motion of the lungs "the flywheel that sets the other forces of the body in motion." Even the simplest life forms expand and contract as they breathe. As we humans live and grow, environmental factors such as stress, ideas about body image, and parental imitation can cause us to lose touch with this life supporting movement pattern. Constantly contracting the belly restricts the diaphragm, deadening the primary respiratory muscles in the abdomen and causing shallow breathing. This in turn restricts the flow of prana to the vital organs, limbs, and nervous system and hampers the natural breathing movements in the abdomen that massage our vital organs.

When I began working with Donna Farhi in 1993, I realized that my most critical work lay in returning to natural abdominal breathing. For the next ten years, I focused my pranayama practice on dismantling my chest-breathing habit—exchanging my unhealthy, restrictive pattern for a more efficient, life-supporting pattern. My asana practice was the laboratory for this exploration. At Donna's urging, I began relaxing my body around my breath, allowing the poses to serve deep breathing.

Up until then, I had given the asana primacy, creating the pose and making my breath conform to it. I began instead to allow my poses to conform to a healthy, abdominal breathing pattern, moving into each asana only as far as I could continue to breathe freely. I began allowing my asanas to oscillate, to evolve. No longer were my asanas stone statues of perceived perfection. They became living, breathing, often surprising, living processes. Instead of bolstering my ego's idea of "good yoga," they now replenished my prana.

In my asana practice, I relax my body around the internal oscillation of my breath, so that the inner breath movement and outer manifestation of my asana fall into synch. When I give full breathing primacy in asana, my mind becomes more present with the experience, rather than running down its long list of parameters for a "perfect" pose. The practice then unifies my body and mind. I no longer do the pose; I become the pose. When I practice in this way, mastery, as defined by Sutra II.47—all effort relaxed and the mind absorbed in the Infinite—naturally occurs.

Because many of us have layered one or more unnatural patterns over our natural breathing pattern, before adding new techniques to our repertoire we must first dismantle our acquired habits so we can use the natural breath as our starting point. Donna Farhi's Breathing Book has been essential in helping me understand the physiology of breathing and common unhealthy breathing habits. It offers exercises to support a return to the natural breathing pattern that is the foundation for pranayama.

After years of exploration into uncovering my natural breath, I've begun to explore simple yogic breathing techniques. Offering these techniques is outside the scope of this book, but I encourage you to find a knowledgeable teacher with a regular asana and pranayama practice to guide you. Pranayama aims to reconnect us with our innate ability to manifest and spread prana throughout our bodies in a skillful and intentional way. Beginning with our unadulterated, essential breath, we can learn to refine breathing patterns further to help bring about the settled mind.

The breath and the mind are intimately linked. This concept is not as esoteric as it might sound. It becomes quite tangible when we are mindful of our breathing and its effect on our mental processes—as well as the mind's reciprocal influence on our respiratory patterns. When the breath is erratic, so are the movements of the mind. When we slow the breath, the mind becomes calm. When the mind becomes intensely concentrated, the breath often almost disappears.

Pay attention to the quality of your breathing when you are angry, sad, content, anxious, afraid, calm, or joyful. How many times has a friend advised you to "take a deep breath" when something has upset you? What happens to your mind when you deepen and slow your breathing?

Often when my mind becomes concentrated while meditating or focused on a project, my breathing almost stops. The first time I noticed this was while on a retreat early in my practice. My body was absolutely motionless, quite upright, even though I was using no muscular energy to remain so. My breathing became extremely shallow, almost nonexistent. Inhalations and exhalations were miniscule blips of movement and occurred only after long intervals of suspension. While I felt perfectly calm as I noted the shallow infrequency of my breathing, my mind would occasionally intrude with the idea that I really ought to take a breath, even though my body did not seem to need it.

What was happening is that the days and weeks of moving slowly, maintaining silence, and building concentration had preserved my vital energy to a point where accumulated prana was literally holding me up internally, without my having to use muscular energy to keep my body erect. Because of the buildup of prana, my body needed less oxygen to maintain its energy level. Thus my respiratory rate slowed. At the same time, my mind was completely still and intensely focused.

Sutra II.51 (Shearer) states, "The fourth kind of pranayama takes us beyond the domain of inner and outer." While none of the sutra translations I've read explain exactly what this fourth type of pranayama is, my interpretation is that it is the slowing of the breath that is interlinked with deep concentration. The next two sutras align with this understanding. Sutra II.52 says, "Then the light of the intellect is unveiled." Sutra II.53 follows: "And the mind is prepared for steadiness." As pranayama practice steadies and refines the breath, the mind lightens, slows its chatter, and becomes more settled. Concentration (dharana) follows.

In the scheme of the eight limbs, Patanjali places pranayama between the externally oriented practices (yama, niyama, and asana) and the subsequent practices of pratyahara, dharana, dhyana, and samadhi for a sound reason. Yama and niyama practice bring peace of mind and order to our lives. Asana practice clears the energy channels in the body to make room for the spread of prana throughout. Pranayama practices replenish the energies we spend in our daily lives, slow the movements of the mind, and balance the nervous system, laying the ground for the settling of the mind. Hatha yoga is the marriage of asana and pranayama. When we've balanced our relationships, environment, and our physical, mental, and emotional bodies through the first four limbs, we are ripe for the development of pratayahara, dharana, dhyana, and samadhi.

Our breath is a metaphor for the natural balancing movements of our lives. Our inhalations are symbolic of all that we continually receive from the world around us. When we inhale, we take in the bounty the world has to offer—not only oxygen but also gifts of love, wisdom, and understanding. Our exhalations express aparigraha, the act of letting go and giving back. When we exhale, we release carbon dioxide, and we contribute our love and wisdom to the collective cache of universal knowledge. In the silent space after the exhalation, we stop and integrate what we've learned. The natural phases of the breath—inhalation, exhalation, and the pause in between—are worthy of years of investigation. First be mindful of your breathing. Then let pranayama practice gradually expand your life energy and settle your mind.

Pranayama in Asana Practice

Allow your asanas to arise from the internal movement of your breath. Rather than performing a pose and making the breath conform to the asana, let your pose evolve as you breathe. In every asana, each inhale and exhale creates either a retractive or a deepening effect. Practice asana so that you allow your body to respond naturally to these movements. Yoga poses are not meant to be static. Keeping your asana alive and moving supports the flow of prana.

Choose a simple forward bend such as Uttanasana (Standing Forward Bend) or Paschimottanasana (Seated Forward Bend). Find your edge, and then back off slightly, so there is more freedom for the body to move within the pose. Feel the breath expanding into your back, and notice how your back wants to lift a bit out of the asana as you inhale (the retractive phase of the breath). As you exhale, feel the body releasing more completely into the forward bend (the deepening phase). Allow your asana to evolve with this oscillating movement, so your body moves more deeply into the pose as the breath allows. Remember that deepening does not necessarily mean moving farther into your image of a perfect pose. Rather, you relax more deeply into your asana as it is. Remain open to how your pose might evolve.

Apply this practice to all your asanas, so the internal movement and external manifestation of each pose are in harmony with each other. Notice the quality of your mind when you practice in this way.

Reflections

■ Get to know your own breathing pattern before you embark on pranayama practice. I highly recommend Donna Farhi's *Breathing Book* as an essential reference for learning proper breathing.

Here's a simple exercise I learned from that book: Lie on your back with the soles of your feet on the floor and your knees bent. Adjust the position of your feet relative to each other and relative to your hips, so the legs feel relaxed. You should not feel as if you have to apply muscular effort to keep your legs upright. Breathe normally. Place one hand on your abdomen and one on your chest. As you inhale, which expands more, your chest or your abdomen? Do you feel your shoulders lift? As you exhale, where do you feel your trunk deflate, in the chest or in the abdomen? Does your breath feel shallow or deep? Time your breathing. How many normal breaths do you take in a minute's time? (Twelve to fifteen breaths per minute is normal.)

This exercise helps you get to know your own propensities. *The Breathing Book* can help you identify your own personal breathing pattern and offers a plethora of explorations and exercises that can help you return to your essential breath.

■ If you find that your normal pattern is to breathe abdominally and you'd like to begin a simple breathing practice, try this one. Lie or sit in a comfortable position so your abdominal muscles are relaxed. Exhale all your breath, so the abdomen becomes concave. Inhale fully, and count the length of your inhalation. Draw out your next exhalation, so it is slightly longer than your inhalation. Again exhale completely. Exhaling completely greatly reduces the amount of CO_2 accumulated in the alveoli, the tiny air sacs inside the lungs, allowing for a greater volume of air to be inhaled. Emptying the lungs also helps rid the body of accumulated toxins.

Lengthening the exhalation slows down the heartbeat due to a physiological phenomenon called sinus arrhythmia, which concerns the relationship between the respiratory and heart rates. When you inhale, the breath quickens slightly; when you exhale, it slows. So when you lengthen your exhalation, your heart rests for a longer time. This breathing practice can help calm your nervous system and increase the intake of prana.

You can begin this practice with a three-minute session. Count the number of breaths you take in the first minute of practice, and compare it to the number of breaths you take in the last minute. Over time you can increase the length of your practice to ten minutes or more. After you finish, sit for a few minutes noting the state of your mind, body, and breath.

It can be helpful to keep a notebook tracking your experiences. Note how you feel in your subsequent daily activities. Note how your breathing changes over time. Since it calms the heartbeat and nervous system, this is an excellent practice to do to prepare you for sleep.

■ Dedicate one day a week, a half day a week, or up to an hour each day to replenishing your prana. At these times, move only minimally. Do not talk; turn off the phone if necessary. Spend at least a few minutes of this time slowing and deepening your breath. You can do this while lying down, if your life has been particularly hectic. Mornings and evenings are best. Choose times when family members are least likely to need you—after they've gone to bed or before they awaken in the morning.

If you are raising a family, these times of building up your prana are absolutely essential. Mothers often become guilt-ridden at the thought of doing something for themselves. This view ultimately brings burnout and results in resentment. You cannot give energy to your family if you've depleted all your prana. Replenishing your life force is not selfish!

It's a matter of survival. It can make the difference between trudging through your daily activities and meeting them with a sense of joy.

■ Practice mindfulness of breathing. As you sit, or as you practice Savasana (Relaxation Pose) at the end of your asana practice, set your intention to be fully mindful of all the phases of your natural breath—inhalation, exhalation, and the pause in between. Note if there is a particular phase of the breath when the mind is more likely to wander. Note if you find it difficult to pay attention to the breath without controlling its depth or rhythm. Pay special attention to the pause between the breaths. What physical sensations arise? What is the character of the mind in this pause? How might your body–mind benefit from relaxing into the pause?

The Fifth Limb: Pratyahara
Detaching from the Senses

20

I'VE TAUGHT YOGA at the First Unitarian Church in Salt Lake City since 1986. Eliot Hall, a spacious, bright room with a maple wood floor, serves as a gracious gathering place for countless community activities. It's a yoga space, a contra dance hall, a meeting place for numerous nonprofit groups, and the site of Salt Lake's most venerable coffeehouse for more than thirty years. The accumulated energies of this longstanding tradition of welcoming the community make for a warm and friendly atmosphere.

Because such a variety of groups use the space, the activities occasionally overlap. Sometimes the overlap brings an unexpected treat, such as the week not long ago when a young pianist—who garnered the Silver Medal in the Gina Bachauer International Piano Competition the following weekend—practiced Tchaikovsky's famous concerto in the next room.

Occasionally it can be challenging. Such was the case many years ago, when children from the church spent an evening setting up a haunted house directly overhead from one of my yoga classes. To say the activities above were simply noisy would not be giving the haunted house its due. It was cacophonous, replete with elephantine foot stomping, punctuated by shrieks and laughter. After our final relaxation, Ashley, a student who had been practicing yoga for about a year mused, "I didn't relax for one second."

A year later, Ashley happened to be in class again while the haunted house was being assembled upstairs. The noise level was similar to that of the year before. After the final relaxation, I asked Ashley if she had been able to relax. She replied, "You know? I barely noticed the noise."

Ashley had entered into the fifth limb of yoga, *pratyahara*. The intervening year of practice had refined her mind; Ashley no longer needed a pristine environment in order to relax in Savasana (Relaxation Pose). She was able to abide in her calm center, regardless of external circumstances. She did not need to shut out the sound; she was simply not bothered by it.

Savasana is the first place that many yogis experience pratyahara. Once the body is physiologically relaxed, a process that takes twelve to fifteen minutes for most people, the mind begins to recede from its reactivity to sensations in the external environment. Even if you've practiced asana for only a short time, it's quite possible that you've experienced pratyahara. Judith Hanson Lasater describes the experience of pratyahara in Savasana as feeling as if you are at the bottom of a well. In pratyahara, the mind is withdrawn from the external world and turned inward. We can be aware of sensation, but we are no longer disturbed by it.

The amount and intensity of sense stimulation in our living environment seems to have accelerated in recent years. Popular films and television programs have become increasingly more violent and sensational. Many people are constantly hooked up to iPods, their chosen music blaring into their ears at all times. I often hear the thumping of mega-stereos in cars that drive along my street and wonder, if I can hear the music so clearly when I'm outside the car and a hundred feet away, what must it be like for the driver? All this suggests that our sensory palates have become so jaded by overstimulation that we no longer can appreciate subtle sensation. It also suggests a cultural desire to escape our inner landscape.

In themselves, sense stimuli are not problematic. If the settling of the mind were dependent on our never being exposed to noise, none of us would ever get there. Rather, it is our response to stimuli that either supports or obscures pratyahara. We can never completely isolate ourselves from the world of sight, sound, touch, taste, and smell, nor would we want to. What pratyahara practice teaches is how to be in the world but not of it.

Ajahn Amaro tells a story of the late forest monk Ajahn Chah, who once found himself annoyed by a festival celebration in the village below his mountain retreat. While trying to meditate, he instead speculated about all the bad karma the villagers were generating by disturbing his meditation.

Noticing his complaining mind, he realized that while the villagers were having a good time, he was simply making himself miserable. He had this insight: "Oh, the sound is just the sound. It's me who is going out to annoy it. If I leave the sound alone, it won't annoy me. It's just doing what it has to do. That's what sound does. It makes sound. This is its job. So if I don't go out and bother the sound, it's not going to bother me. Aha!"

In this realization is the essence of pratyahara. Sensation itself is not a problem. Even in the quietest, most serene environment, our minds can easily be disturbed. It is our reactions to sensation that create mental unrest. In pratyahara, we withdraw our attachment and aversion to the delights and irritations of the senses.

Pratyahara lies at a major intersection of the eight limbs. Both previous and subsequent limbs feed its evolution. Niyamas such as saucha, which helps refine our sensory palate, santosha, which conditions us to be content with our present reality, and tapas, in which we simplify, naturally removing some of the superfluous stimuli in our lives, begin the process of detachment. Mindful practice of asana further refines our physical awareness. As we develop the ability to remain at our edge in poses that present difficulty, our reflexive reactivity to unpleasant sensation begins to fade. Dharana, the sixth limb, collects our mind onto a single object, relinquishing all other objects to the background.

Two sutras, II.54 and II.55, describe the experience of pratyahara. Shearer translates II.54 as: "The senses retire from their objects by following the natural inward movement of the mind." II.55 says, "From this comes supreme mastery of the senses." Shearer's translation of Sutra II.53 (on the result of pranayama practice) says, "And the mind is prepared for steadiness." From this we might conclude that, as pranayama helps the mind to settle and become more concentrated, the natural movement of mind shifts from the external to the internal.

Often translated as "withdrawal from the senses," pratyahara is the beginning of the mind's intentional movement inward. I've found the idea of withdrawal from the senses problematic, in that this definition seems to imply a purposeful isolation from the external world. This seems tantamount to denying reality. For most of us practicing yoga in the West, the mundane activities of our daily lives provide fertile ground for practice.

Pratyahara has developed in my own practice not by withdrawing myself from the world of the senses but rather by becoming acutely aware of this fascinating realm. Looking directly at sensation and seeing its inherently impermanent and insubstantial nature has allowed my attachment to it to melt away naturally, without resistance.

As a lifelong musician, hearing is probably the best developed of my senses. Because of my conditioning as a musician, music can distract me far more easily than most other sensations. While the students in my class could simply enjoy the sounds of the Gina Bachauer finalist practicing during our asana classes, my mind was swept up in an analytical frenzy. I noted the pianist's subtle phrasing and his stellar left hand technique. I even mentally inserted familiar oboe parts into the appropriate places as he practiced his concerto. While my students could easily hear the pianist as excellent background music, my mind went crazy. The pianist was truly extraordinary, and although I enjoyed hearing him practice, it was difficult for me to detach myself from my own conditioning and allow the sound to recede into the background.

Knowing that what I hear can easily distract me, "hearing meditation" has been an excellent practice for me in developing pratyahara. I learned it about ten years ago while on retreat. The late afternoon walking meditation that takes place just before dinnertime has always been a challenging time for me. Perhaps it's caused by anticipation of the sense pleasures to come at dinnertime, or maybe the hour between 4:00 and 5:00 is simply a time when my mind naturally descends into entropy. Regardless of the cause, my mind always behaves a bit like a pinball at this time of day, bouncing from thought to thought, sensation to sensation, unable to adhere to anything.

During one frustrating session, I wondered if the movement of walking might actually aggravate my already overstimulated mind. I stopped on the walking path, closed my eyes, and stood quietly. Free from the responsibility of trying to pin down the sensations of walking, my mind immediately turned to the sense of hearing. The rustling of treetops in the breeze, cars driving along the distant highway, the scrambling of chipmunks, power tools growling at a construction site down the road, the clanking of pans being washed in the kitchen—all these sounds became my world. I noted how and where the timbre of each sound resonated in my body. I noted my tendency to label some sounds as pleasant and others as unpleasant and my attendant responses of attachment and aversion. I noted the constantly changing nature of this sonic feast. My entire being became subsumed by the sounds in my environment.

I practiced this meditation each day for the remainder of the retreat. Over time, the sounds themselves ceased to matter. Awareness, the settled mind, simply knew the sounds but was no longer reactive to them. A still, unbiased awareness emerged into the foreground, replacing the sounds that had previously consumed me. The sounds were still there, but they no longer ruled me. By moving fully into my most distractible sense store, I was able to detach myself from it and settle into pratyahara. I believe this is what Sutra II.55 means by "mastery of the senses."

In practicing hearing meditation, I employed what the Buddha called the four foundations of mindfulness. These foundations are simply ways of connecting with the present moment. The foundations include all the various avenues through which we relate to our experience. All the foundations are interdependent; in cultivating any single area, all the others are strengthened. Often several or all of them can come into play simultaneously. To practice using this model, you let the mind turn to whichever foundation is most predominant at the time. Here's how it works:

The first foundation is mindfulness of the body. When we practice mindfulness of the sensations of sitting, walking, lying, standing, and breathing, we are practicing mindfulness of the body. Being mindful of the experience of the senses is another aspect of the first foundation. When a sound, sight, taste, smell, or felt sensation becomes predominant in our experience, we direct our mind toward it. Rather than seeing body sensation as a distraction, we investigate it. The sensation becomes our meditation. In my hearing meditations, I became aware of the sounds in the environment and how different sounds resonated within my body.

Asana practice provides an excellent opportunity to explore mindfulness of the body. We allow our minds to investigate the sensations that are either most predominant or most interesting. As the mind becomes absorbed in a sensation, we begin to discover aspects of it that we previously may not have understood—most important, its impermanent and

constantly changing nature. Instead of moving quickly through our practice, flitting from one pose to the next, we slow down, spending whatever
time is necessary to allow us to investigate the arising sensations. We watch
how sensations evolve. By exploring the sensations we feel at our edge, we
begin to understand their impermanent nature and thus become less reactive to them.

The second foundation of mindfulness is called mindfulness of feeling.
In this context, feeling refers not to emotions but our felt interpretation of
a sensation. In the second foundation, we note whether we categorize a
sensation as pleasant, unpleasant, or neutral. This foundation is a crucial
link to understanding our relationship to sensations, and it allows us to
unhook ourselves from reactivity and judging.

When we categorize a sensation as pleasant, we are likely to want to cling
to it. When we find a sensation to be unpleasant, we respond to it with
aversion. When a sensation feels neutral, we tend to lose interest altogether.
In my hearing meditations, I noted my preference for some sounds, usually the sounds I considered to be natural elements, such as the wind and
the scrambling chipmunks, over other sounds that I deemed unnatural,
such as the sounds of car motors or construction work.

In noting the feeling nature of each sensation, we can change patterns
of reactivity at an elemental level. The most basic of these patterns are crav-
ing, aversion, and ignorance—not coincidentally the qualities the Buddha
called the root of all suffering. When we note that we perceive a sensation
to be pleasant, unpleasant, or neutral, we can make a choice about how to
respond. We no longer have to respond automatically to pleasant sensation
by clinging to it, to unpleasant sensation by trying to push it away, or to
neutral sensation by spacing out. We can simply investigate each sensation
as it arises, without having to react to it. Our minds experience each sensation, without becoming disturbed by it. This is the essence of pratyahara.

The third foundation is mindfulness of mental states. In this foundation,
we note mental states, such as whether the mind is calm, concentrated, or
distracted, and whatever emotions might be present. Mindfulness of mental states also includes noting responses of attachment or aversion, so in
this way the third foundation is closely linked to the second.

In my hearing meditation, I used the third foundation to note my mental/emotional response to the sounds I enjoyed and the ones I didn't like. I found that it made no difference whether I wished the power tools would stop or whether I loved the sound of the breeze. The power tools would continue until their services were no longer required, and I certainly could not control the wind. My choice became simply to note it all. My opinions made not a whit of difference except to me, and for me they mostly produced agitation.

Because we filter much of our experience through the veil of our emotions, mindfulness of the third foundation is crucial to freeing us from reactivity. While being mindful of mental/emotional states, we do not try to change them; we simply seek to understand them. When we are experiencing a powerful emotion, it is helpful to feel where and how that emotion resides in the body (mindfulness of the body). As with the first foundation, when we explore the felt sense of our emotions, we experience their changing nature. We become less identified with them because they no longer feel so solid and impenetrable. Again, this leads us into pratyahara.

The fourth foundation arises naturally as we practice the others. This foundation is called mindfulness of the dharma. Mindfulness of the dharma is the awareness of the impermanent and therefore ultimately unsatisfying nature of all sensation. When we delve deeply into the sensations we feel, we ultimately discover that they are not so solid as we thought when we simply looked at their surface. We discover that because of their impermanent nature, we in fact cannot define ourselves by them. Nor is it necessary to try to push them away, since they will eventually disappear or morph into something else. Again, here we find the essence of pratyahara. We are fully aware of the world of sensation but no longer disturbed by it.

Practicing the foundations, and therefore pratyahara, helps us to see for ourselves that our happiness or unhappiness does not depend on what is happening in the external world. Wonderful experiences, great wealth, enduring relationships can certainly give momentary pleasure. And there is nothing wrong with experiencing pleasure, as long as we know that the accumulation of pleasures cannot bring lasting happiness.

Practicing pratyahara helps us to see the pleasure inherent in the settled mind, the mind that is not pulled hither and yon by the fleeting pleasures and pains of the ever-changing external world.

Pratyahara in Asana Practice

When you can, give yourself twenty minutes for Savasana. In order for pratyahara to arise in Savasana, it is helpful for the nervous system to be relaxed. Because it takes the body twelve to fifteen minutes to achieve physical relaxation, a short Savasana does not necessarily support pratyahara. You might begin Savasana by practicing a minute or two of hearing meditation.

Allowing asana to arise from the oscillating movements of the breath, as described in the previous chapter, helps relax the body–mind, so you can shift more easily into pratyahara. As this way of practicing becomes integrated and you no longer have to think about it (unconscious competence), pratyahara can arise within each asana as well.

Reflections

- Sitting quietly in nature and experiencing its myriad sensations can help develop pratyahara. Make a practice of spending time outside on a regular basis. Commit to visiting a state or national park or a green space once a week, or simply relax in your backyard. Although, if you're like me, sitting in your backyard may cause your mind to obsess about all the yard work you need to do!

  If hearing is a strong sense for you, practice hearing meditation. Do not reach out for sound; allow the sound to come to you (because it will come to you anyway). The extra effort is not necessary.

  If touch is your sensation, close your eyes and feel the ground beneath your feet, the sun or wind on your skin. Perhaps you are especially sensitive to heat or cold. Can you allow yourself to be present with heat or cold, to feel the actual sensation of heat and cold without contracting away from it?

  If seeing is your sense, focus on a patch of ground and watch the activity of small animals, insects, and birds. Or watch the clouds moving through the sky. Experiment with diffusing your vision, allowing your eyes to recede so that you are not focusing on anything in particular. Do not reach out with the eyes; let visual sensation come to you.

If your sense of smell is strong, sit and focus on the fragrances in the air. The sense of smell seems particularly susceptible to forming preferences. Which smells do you like and which do you dislike?

If you are especially attracted to taste, practice eating meditation. Bring along a piece of fruit to eat slowly and mindfully, feeling the texture and taste.

Rivers and streams are excellent places to experience changing sensations in the realms of hearing, seeing, touch and smell.

Note which of the four foundations is predominant. Be mindful of the body, feeling quality, mental/emotional response, or changing nature, depending on what you feel most strongly. Note if the predominance of the foundations shifts from week to week, or if your mind wants to explore more than one foundation.

■ Practice the four foundations in asana practice. Choose a pose you like and one you do not like. Move into each pose to your intelligent edge—the place where you feel sensation but can still breathe easily. Stay for five minutes, focusing your mind on the sensations that arise. Watch the evolution of these sensations and note your responses to them.

Make sure you choose poses that are possible to remain in for a while. For example, even if you love or cannot stand to practice arm balances or Virabhadrasana II (Warrior Pose II), it's probably better not to try to hold them for five minutes. Seated, supine, or prone positions are best for this exploration.

The Sixth Limb: Dharana
Collecting the Mind

21

W HEN I WAS in college, a friend and I took a basic drawing class together. The teacher was quite inspiring, and I looked forward to the class each week. My admiration for the teacher prompted me to be uncharacteristically enthusiastic about completing assignments, sometimes even going out of my way to do more than was required—a pattern that was not my norm at the time.

One evening, my classmate set up a still life at his house for us to render in charcoal. When we finished drawing, I was amazed that three hours had passed. During that time, I had not left my drawing, physically or mentally. I remembered nothing about my time at the easel. My only proof that I had accomplished anything was a dramatic, almost animated rendering of our inanimate setup.

The experience was immensely satisfying, partly because it produced a lively and beautiful drawing, but even more so because my concentration on the project was so complete. I had collected my energies on my drawing so utterly that my usual mental wanderings had disappeared—or at least had become inconsequential compared with the project at hand.

For many years, having an enjoyable project to focus on was my vehicle for accessing the quality of *dharana*, or concentration, the sixth of Patanjali's eight limbs. Dharana is the first of the three limbs that Alistair Shearer calls the "heart of yoga." The sixth, seventh, and eighth limbs are concerned with turning the mind inward and the eventual complete settling of the mind. Quite often the three blur together, as I believe they did during my drawing project. In this and the two chapters that follow, I will attempt to draw distinctions among these three limbs, the limbs that are most directly concerned with the refinement of consciousness.

Dharana is the collecting of the mind onto a particular object—usually a mantra, a physical object such as a candle, a concept or quality you'd like to develop, or the breath. As we gather the mind's disparate energies onto a single object, we begin to isolate the mind from its normal wanderings. When we begin practicing dharana, it is helpful to remember that most of us have spent most of our lives allowing our minds to run out of control. The momentum toward mental entropy is rather like that of a runaway train.

Because of this, this stage of practice is characterized by heroic effort. When we sit down to practice dharana, our minds can slip off our object of concentration hundreds of times within a short period. This can become very frustrating. However, it is helpful to note that the simple fact that we have noticed the chaos in the mind is a sign that we're moving in the direction of greater awareness. If we are not purposely paying attention, the monkey mind does not seem out of the ordinary. Knowing that the mind is out of control shows that we are becoming more aware. Each of the hundreds of times we bring the mind back to its object strengthens our practice of dharana.

When we practice dharana, we gather our attention onto our chosen object and let go of all that is not the object. When I was in Italy during college, I was especially fascinated by Michelangelo's unfinished sculptures, figures that appear to be emerging from a block of marble. In creating his sculptures, Michelangelo chipped away everything that was not essential to the figure. What emerged was a precise representation of his original intention.

In practicing dharana, this is what we are doing—letting go of everything that is not the object of our meditation. In this way, concentration practice and pratyahara practice are interwoven. Pratyahara teaches us to let go of attachment to sense experiences. In dharana, sense stimuli naturally fall away as we collect our energies onto a central object.

When I first began vipassana practice, I did not find the primary object— my breath—nearly as engrossing as I had found the art projects or piano sonatas of my past. I was, in fact, much more drawn to the myriad dramas stampeding through my mind—the thoughts and my mental/emotional reactions to them. With time and perseverance, my mind gradually began to enjoy being concentrated. The satisfaction derived from a peaceful mind was far greater than the extreme highs and lows I experienced when I was caught up in the drama.

There are two components to developing dharana. These are: aiming the mind toward an object of concentration and sustaining the attention on the object. The Pali word for aiming the mind is *vitaca*. Vitaca is the initial intention to aim the mind in the direction of the primary object of concentration. Traditional objects include the breath, a mantra, or a concept or quality we'd like to develop, such as *metta* (translated from Pali as "loving kindness" or "friendship"). When we practice vitaca, we corral the mind back to the object once we realize it has strayed.

The sustaining phase of dharana is called *vicara*. Vicara is described as "rubbing the object" with our attention. Once we have brought the mind back to the object, rather than having it bounce right off again and go back to its wanderings, we endeavor to adhere the mind to the object. This is vicara. Both phases of concentration are needed in order to steady the mind.

Because I am most familiar with using the breath as my primary object during sitting meditation and the sensations in my feet during walking meditation, I will focus dharana instructions on just these two objects. Of course, if your dharana practice also includes mantras, visualizations, or daily life practices, you can apply the following techniques to whatever you choose.

In sitting meditation, begin by setting yourself up in a comfortable sitting position. This may require some trial and error, as you figure out which position best supports a healthy spine and the quieting of your mind. I began years ago sitting on a meditation bench. Four years into practice I shifted to sitting on folded blankets, and for the past ten years I've enjoyed sitting on a V-shaped cushion. If your hips, quadriceps, hamstrings, or knees restrict your ability to sit on the floor, you may find sitting in a chair to be the best option.

Remember that even a cushy recliner is not going to be 100 percent comfortable if you are sitting for a long period of time. So experiment with your sitting position as long as you need to, but know that discomfort may arise. This is not a sign that something is wrong with your practice. Rather, the aches and pains you experience may simply be signs that your awareness has sharpened and you are feeling sensations that were previously submerged.

As you sit, become aware of your breathing. Note where you feel the breath most clearly in the body. The breath awareness practice in chapter is helpful here. Most people tend to feel their breath most clearly in the nostrils or in the rising and falling of the abdomen, although I've often found the sensation of the breath passing through my throat to be interesting. Choose a place, and begin to feel the sensation of your breath there. Aim your mind toward the sensation (vitaca). After you have made contact with the breath, sustain the attention on those sensations (vicara).

The most helpful instruction I've heard in developing dharana is this: Avoid the tendency to commit to more than the mind is capable of doing. If you commit to sitting for twenty minutes with unwavering concentration, you will likely be disappointed within a breath or two. After a few forays into fantasy, you may be tempted to give up. Because you are teaching your mind a new skill, one that is likely the opposite of your mind's well-cultivated habits, it is highly unlikely that you will be able to sustain concentration for very long at first. Commit to being aware of just this present inhalation, then just this exhalation, then just this still space. As each part of the breath arises, aim and then sustain the mind in its direction. Over time, through continued practice, a continuity of awareness will develop.

This is not to say that the mind will not wander as you practice this way. It will. This process is like learning any skill. When I'm trying to make my fingers adapt to a difficult passage on my oboe, I break down the phrase into sections. I practice each section until my fingers are facile. Then I move on to the next section. When I'm able to play each section cleanly, I string the sections together, smoothing out the transitions between them. In the same way, you teach the mind to behave in a way that is radically different from its usual out-of-control condition by breaking down each part of your object of concentration. It is painstaking work, but it builds a solid foundation for collecting the mind.

To practice walking meditation, choose a place to walk, indoors or outdoors. Choose a pathway between two landmarks, perhaps between two trees or the length of a hallway. Begin walking back and forth along your path. Start walking slightly more slowly than your normal pace. For now, simply be aware of the motion of your legs. Mentally note "left, right, left, right." Gradually slow your pace, and look more closely at the components of each step, becoming aware of lifting the foot, moving it, and then placing it on the ground.

Your gait may slow to almost a snail's pace, where it may take a minute or two to walk one length of your path. At that point, you can become aware of more intricate details—the sensation of weight shifting from the heel to the toe of the back foot, the point where the foot lifts off the ground, the sensation of the foot gliding through the air, the initial contact of the heel with the ground, and the feeling of weight shifting across to the ball of the foot. Again, you can apply the concepts of vitaca and vicara to each component of each step.

I initially found walking meditation much easier than sitting. That may be because I was raised in a family that enjoyed walking, but it could also be because the sensations of walking are not quite so subtle as those of the breath. I also love walking meditation because it has taught me how to be mindful at times other than when I am sitting on my meditation cushion. Walking meditation provides a bridge between formal practice and mindfulness of daily activities.

So far I've written a lot about the effort required to develop dharana. Of course, effort and commitment are absolutely necessary. When our minds become more concentrated, however, they become not only quite steady but also relaxed and profoundly peaceful. Far from my former image of concentration as a person sitting with furrowed brow, straining hard to focus on a particular object, when dharana is developed it brings great happiness and spaciousness to the mind.

Concentration brings relief from the chaos of the mind. As we build dharana, the energies normally dissipated through rampant fantasy become more collected. In this way, we also build prana by practicing dharana. Cultivating concentration steadies the mind so it can open itself to wisdom practice, dhyana (meditation, the seventh limb).

According to Buddhist thought, the proximate cause for the development of concentration is happiness. In terms of the eight limbs, happiness arises as a result of right action or practicing ethical behavior (such as the yamas). Whereas unskillful behavior creates agitation and anxiety about the repercussions of our actions, ethical behavior creates the conditions necessary for peace of mind.

Dharana can be practiced in many ways. It is said that the Buddha identified forty various objects of concentration that he assigned to his monks, depending on where they needed balance. For example, a monk with angry or hostile tendencies would be given the practice of the first brahma-vihara—metta (loving kindness or friendship). Metta practice develops both concentration and the quality of good will, thus balancing the tendency toward ill will.

I've focused a great deal of my practice on the development of metta. If you find yourself drawn to this practice, I recommend that you read Lovingkindness: The Revolutionary Art of Happiness by Sharon Salzberg. Practicing metta has been a powerful tool for developing mental steadiness in my practice. Because I do not feel that my writing a few paragraphs about metta would come close to doing justice to such an important practice, I will not elaborate here. What is important to understand about this and other brahma-vihara practices (which include compassion, joy, and equanimity) is that dharana practice has implications far beyond simply steadying our minds. Through these practices we develop not only steadiness of mind but lovely mental qualities that help us live more peacefully.

Wherever we choose to focus our minds, we plant seeds. The more time we spend watering, feeding, and caring for these seeds, the stronger they will grow. If we plant and cultivate seeds of kindness, the resulting tree will be benevolent. If we plant and cultivate seeds of anger, the resulting tree will be hostile.

Dharana practice gives us our first window into what our minds spend their energy cultivating. Sometimes the thoughts we find ourselves replaying over and over are not what we, in our heart of hearts, would really want to see grow into a huge tree. It is at this level where we can begin to make a choice. I believe this is the greatest power we have. We can choose to be jerked about by the monkey that's been left in charge of our undisciplined minds, or we can choose to tame that monkey so that we can put him to work in ways that enrich our lives and the lives of those around us.

Dharana in Your Asana Practice

Use your asana practice as an opportunity to practice dharana. Even though the mind is often lost in thoughts of the present or future, our bodies are always in the present. Using the sensations of asana as an object of concentration brings us right into the present moment. The judgments and analyses your mind creates around asana practice are extra and are not reflective of the present. Let these go, and simply be present with your practice.

Reflections

■ Use the first of the four foundations of mindfulness (mindfulness of the body) to direct and refine your dharana practice. For example, if you are focusing on your breath, feel the sensations of the breath in the area of your body where your breath feels clearest. In walking meditation, direct your mindfulness to the sensations you feel in the legs and feet. Other foundations of mindfulness may also appear. Note these as well. The foundations give your mind a concrete place to focus.

■ Much as we can use our senses to develop pratyahara, we can use them to develop dharana. Choose an object—a flower, a stone, a work of art, a piece of driftwood. Study your object, feeling its texture and weight, looking at its color and form. Spend some time, at least five to ten minutes or more. Note the quality of your mind as you study your object. Take time to be with your object of attention regularly. Note how your relationship with it evolves over time.

■ Commit to whatever amount of practice is practical for your life. If sitting five minutes upon arising or before going to bed is doable, consider yourself fortunate! Committing to accomplishing one of your daily tasks with complete attention is a wonderful practice as well. Think about how you can expand concentration practice into your life.

The Seventh Limb: 22
Dhyana: Witnessing Presence

A YEAR AFTER my first meditation retreat, I attended another, this time for ten days. In the first few days, I was surprised and disappointed to note that keeping my mind on the breath was no less of a struggle than it had been a year before, despite the fact that I had practiced faithfully all year. Hundreds of times each day, my mind wandered off; hundreds of times, I brought it back to the breath. Mental enticements—fantasies great and small—changed from time to time, but my mind's fierce addiction to them remained quite steady. The breath was just not as compelling as my mind-made drama.

Nonetheless I persevered, constantly corralling the wild monkey back to the breath. One afternoon, about a week into the retreat, I was startled to note a new development. I was able to watch my mind wandering off and bringing itself back to the breath. I was no longer directing the process. I could sit back and witness the entire show—the passing of all the fantasies, physical sensations, and mental states, all interwoven with my breathing—without becoming identified. The thousands of times I had brought my mind back to the breath (dharana) had shifted my mind's momentum. The stream of consciousness was now continuous and no longer needed me to control things. This was *dhyana*, the seventh of the eight limbs.

It is here, at the junction of dharana and dhyana, where distinctions begin to blur. Dharana, dhyana, and samadhi are often experienced simultaneously. When dhyana occurs, dharana is usually present. Samadhi arises within the simultaneous occurrence of dharana and dhyana. Distinctions are subtle indeed. In the sutras, the three are called *samyana*, or "perfect discipline."

When we concentrate on a particular object, as in dharana, we aim our attention in its direction and sustain that attention on the object. In dhyana, when concentration becomes continuous, we witness the object unobstructed by the layers of our conditioning and subjectivity. From this, wisdom develops.

Alistair Shearer distinguishes dharana and dhyana in this way: Sutra III.1: "When the attention is held focused on an object, this is known as dharana." Sutra III.2: "When awareness flows evenly toward the point of attention, this is known as dhyana."

In chapter 21, I wrote about the experience of concentration as it related to an art project. In reality, dharana was not the only limb at work there. The initial directing of my mind toward drawing developed concentration in my mind. As time passed, I was able to witness the drawing coming to life. My hands held the charcoal and marked the page, but I was no longer directing the show. All my drawing practice over the years allowed the process to become automatic. In essence, the years of focusing my attention (dharana) on learning how to draw bore its fruits in my ability to let go of the techniques I'd learned and simply allow those techniques to play themselves through me (dhyana). (This also conforms to the "conscious competence" model outlined in chapter 3. At this stage in my drawing practice, I had moved into unconscious competence.)

The level of profound absorption that allowed me to lose track of time was samadhi. By that time, all three limbs were occurring simultaneously. At this singular point on my life path, I understand dharana, dhyana, and samadhi to be varying degrees of the settled mind, increasingly effortless and profound.

Bernard Bouanchaud describes the meaning of Sutra III.2 this way: "With prolonged focus on one object, concentration becomes meditation, in which the grasp of the object is direct—instantaneous, new, and unforgettable. This interaction between subject and object leaves a deep impression that replaces understanding that is based on memory and the past." The "instantaneous, new, and unforgettable" grasp of an object, free from conditioning of past beliefs about it, describes the experience of what vipassana meditation practitioners call insight.

To illustrate, I'd like to revisit my first-ever meditation retreat and my experience dealing with physical pain. As I already recounted, physical discomfort plus lots of mental whining plunged me into a pretty bitter stew in those first few days. The day of respite following my doorknob experience felt like a well-deserved dessert course. When my mind and body retreated into chaos later on, I was disappointed, but having experienced one satisfying moment of mindfulness, I knew now that there was more to this practice than just enduring one insult after another.

Earlier in the retreat, Pujari had spoken about using physical discomfort as an object for developing mindfulness. I attempted this practice during the first few days, approaching it as a possible means of escape from my discomfort. I thought that perhaps if I looked at the pain, it would go away. That didn't work out as I'd hoped, so I quickly abandoned the practice to indulge in pleasant fantasies.

A few days later, I decided to try again. At that point my knees and back were no longer harassing me, but my shoulder pain was steadily escalating into the red zone. Buoyed this time by my pleasant doorknob experience, I began investigating the sensation in my shoulder. Instead of hoping that concentrating on the pain might make it disappear, I brought a sense of curiosity to the process. I saw the discomfort as it was, a constantly changing symphony of sensation. In reality, the pain had a beginning, middle, and end. It arose subtly, intensified, and gradually vanished at almost regular intervals. Each incidence of shoulder sensation lasted maybe five seconds and then subsided for about five seconds.

Earlier in the retreat, I could not see the physical discomfort in my shoulder so clearly. Even though I'd observed its changing nature, aversion flavored my mental state with such bitterness that my mind was unable to settle. I saw the pain, and I disliked it. I lobbed my consciousness at it, hoping to vanquish it. This time, because I had no agenda, I was able to see clearly into the sensation. In that moment, I saw directly—not theoretically—the constantly changing, impermanent nature of the sensation in my shoulder. I realized in that moment that the evolving nature of my shoulder pain was offering me a view into the impermanent nature of all phenomena.

The realization that my shoulder pain was not solid or permanent initiated a radical shift in my way of being. While I might not enjoy the experience of physical, mental, or emotional pain, I now know unequivocally that whatever I'm experiencing will change. Knowing that allows me to relax into discomfort rather than becoming overwhelmed. Earlier in the retreat, I saw physical discomfort as a defect in my practice. Now I understood that the pain was simply what was happening in the present moment. It was no more or less significant than the pleasant sensations I'd felt reaching for the doorknob. I didn't have to like the pain, but I also didn't have to generate more suffering by hating it.

Just because I experienced that realization does not mean that I have subsequently always met the experience of discomfort—or even the anticipation of possible discomfort—with ease. My conditioning surrounding physical pain is a well-practiced habit, and it sometimes plays itself out in less than skillful ways. This is especially apparent when I feel my fingers digging into the arms of a dentist's chair, often before the dentist has even done anything! Still, there are times when I can relax into the ever-changing process of pleasant and unpleasant physical, mental, and emotional sensation and let it be. The difference now is that I know I have a choice.

Had I not spent several days developing concentration on the breath (dharana), my mind would not have been able to stay with the discomfort in my shoulder long enough for its nature to be revealed. As dharana strengthened, I was able to expand my consciousness outward and delve more deeply into what was present. This mindfulness yielded a direct, undeniable experience of the basic nature of all phenomena: that all things are impermanent.

This is my current understanding of dhyana. When we aim the steadied mind toward the present experience, and the stream of consciousness is continuous, we see the object clearly, unadorned by our preconceptions. From this, wisdom arises.

In his book *Seeking the Heart of Wisdom*, Jack Kornfield refers to the expansion of concentration as "moment-to-moment samadhi." In this practice, we allow the mind to focus on whatever is present. In expanding our awareness from a singular object to include all areas of experience, we develop the ability to still the mind regardless of what is present. Again, some facility in the practice of dharana is necessary for the mind to be able to remain a steady witness to the flurry of phenomena as it parades by.

Dhyana is often defined as "witnessing presence." To be a witness is to observe events simply as they are, without layering judgments or evaluations on top of them. While the habit of judging may be deeply rooted for many of us, with practice the pattern can evolve. As the steadiness of dharana widens into the flow of dhyana, our minds become more impartial. As we witness sensations, thoughts, and mental states simply as they are, we begin to see that no judgment is required. The evaluations we layer over our experience only serve to obscure what is true.

This practice therefore has tremendous implications in our lives. As we dismantle our tendency to judge simple phenomena, such as the breath or our prowess or lack thereof in asana practice, we start to question the truth of our judgments of others as well. These judgments and evaluations to which we so tenaciously cling have the power to inflict unfathomable harm.

In the asana chapter, I wrote about my troubles with my schizoaffective neighbor. While he might have zeroed in on my house as his personal boogeyman no matter what, his father had planted the seeds of his discontent many years before. Sometime before I moved into my house, the father built a chain-link fence between our properties. He was apparently unclear about the location of the property line however, and he placed the fence six inches inside his property line. This means that a six-inch strip of his property extends along the entire length of my side of the fence. It would not be an exaggeration to say that the father reminded me of this, in a very accusing way, more than fifty times over ten years. I always responded by saying if he wanted to move the fence, it was fine with me. Each time he in turn responded by shrugging me off, saying that moving the fence would be too much trouble. So I'm certain that his son was aware that his father saw me as a thief of their property, even though I had nothing to do with where he'd placed the fence. Over time, the story became so real and so horrendous in both of their minds that they both felt compelled to harass me at every opportunity.

Without trying to make my little neighborhood situation sound too grandiose, situations like this one contain the seeds of major conflict— even war. How many wars have been fought over perceived (or misperceived) boundary disputes? How many wars are still being waged over real or imagined injustices that happened hundreds or thousands of years ago? Remember the famous nineteenth-century feuding families, the Hatfields and the McCoys? More than a dozen family members on both sides died as the result of a legendary, decades-long conflict sparked by a dispute over the ownership of a pig. How many factions in the current religious wars have actually experienced some sort of direct negative experience with their so-called enemies? Probably very few, but still the hatred endures. How often have we found our own judgment of someone to be erroneous after spending months or years living in resentment or hatred? All this suffering stems from thoughts and judgments that come from our minds.

One of my favorite Joseph Goldstein quotes is "The thought of your mother is not your mother. The thought of your mother is just a thought." The beliefs that divide us are just thoughts. The prejudices we cling to so fiercely are just opinions, which are just thoughts. And thoughts have no substance. When we observe thoughts from within the perspective of our true mind—the expansive, witnessing presence—we see them as insubstantial and one-dimensional.

The image that has come to me time and again as I rest in the spacious mind of dhyana is that the thoughts that are arising appear to be nothing more than a tape chattering nonsense at high speed, somewhere off in the distance. At these times of dwelling in the settled mind, my thoughts are not at all enticing. They arise, they pass, and they leave no mark.

The situation with my neighbor has been a tremendously challenging practice for me. While I no longer tolerate harassing behavior, I do feel compassion for this person whose suffering is so profound that he feels he must spread it around the neighborhood. Hating my neighbor changes nothing; it only feeds the pattern of hostility.

Feeling compassion does not preclude my taking action, however. When one person's behavior severely lessens the quality of life of many around him, steps must be taken to remedy the situation. This means calling police if I feel threatened by my neighbor's behavior. It means developing a community of solidarity and support with other concerned neighbors. Pujari calls this "ruthless compassion." It comes from seeing the situation clearly and responding in a way that creates the most harmonious solution for everyone involved.

When we enter the state of witnessing, we see clearly into our experience without layering our beliefs and judgments onto it. In this way, we can see our world with all its wonders and horrors, without our minds becoming overwhelmed. This does not mean that we respond with indifference to injustices we observe. When we are able to witness a situation clearly, without judgments and preconceptions, we can approach each problem from a mind of caring and compassion rather than one of anger.

Meditation practice is not about coming to a place where we experience only pleasant thoughts and enjoyable mental states. Rather, as our practice matures, we begin to understand the insubstantiality of the phenomena projected onto the screen of awareness. We are able to meet pleasant and unpleasant thoughts and mental states with equanimity. This witnessing consciousness expands into our daily life practice as well. The practice of dhyana develops clear, unbiased seeing. This clarity is wisdom.

Dhyana in Asana Practice

What poses do you love to practice? Are there poses you dislike? Do you know why you gravitate toward certain asanas and avoid others? Include a pose you dislike in your daily practice. Be attentive to the sensations occurring in the pose, especially those sensations you find uncomfortable. Do you find yourself labeling these sensations as "bad" without really feeling them? Stay in the pose long enough that you can feel the evolution of the unpleasant sensations. (It's best to choose a pose you can hold a while for this exploration. So arm balances might not be your best choice, even if they are your least favorite poses!)

In the discussion of ahimsa, I suggested practicing asana, noting the judgments—positive and negative—that surround your practice. This practice can also support the development of dhyana. These judgments obscure the moment-to-moment experience of asana. Use your skills in dharana (concentration) to be mindful of the physical sensations that accompany each pose. Note your judgments. Note whether these judgments enhance practice or whether they get in the way of seeing practice clearly. Become a witness to these judgments as well. Avoid judging your judgments!

Reflections

■ When your mind feels stable and concentrated from dharana practice, expand your meditation to include whatever sensation is predominant in the moment. Use the four foundations of mindfulness to stabilize your focus. For example, use mindfulness of the body to sense physical sensation or to locate an emotion within your body. Investigate each sensation as it arises. If nothing grabs your attention, return to your breath.

■ Reflect on a situation in your life where there is conflict. What originally caused the rift? In what ways have you expanded that conflict by judging it? Can you separate your ideas about the situation from the reality of it? How does this change your relationship to conflict?

The Eighth Limb
Samadhi: Entering the Timeless

23

OW DOES ONE WRITE about what is beyond words, beyond time and beyond space? At best, it must be accomplished indirectly, through story. Describing *samadhi* is as effective as describing a piece of music. No amount of talking, no matter how eloquent, can substitute for the experience of hearing the music. So I will attempt to describe samadhi by sharing two past events, one fun and fleeting and the other transformational, that illustrate what I believe were samadhi experiences. My hope is that these stories will inspire similar reflections for you.

Early in my life, I studied piano for nine years. While I was not especially dedicated early on, practicing boring scales and rudimentary pieces, once I began playing romantic fare, such as Chopin, Debussy, and Ravel, playing piano took on its own life. More times than I can remember, when I had practiced a particular piece of music enough, I could let go of having to think about fingerings, when to pedal, when to play loudly, or when to soften my touch. At those times, the music would pour through me and move my fingers without my guidance. I was no longer directing the process; it happened completely on its own. At those times, I could play for hours, and it would feel like minutes. I had no sense of being a part of the process. My identity was completely subsumed. There was just music.

Most of us have felt this type of absorption at times in our lives. I have observed it in other musicians, but it is certainly not limited to music or any other particular discipline. Samadhi happens when we let go of ourselves, our constructed identities, and merge with what is present. It can happen any time—when we dance or sing, when we walk in nature, when we wash dishes or sit silently in meditation. I believe that samadhi was also present when I became completely absorbed in my charcoal drawing. At those times when we are no longer bound by the concepts of time and space, we enter samadhi.

According to Alistair Shearer's translation, Sutra III.3 describes samadhi this way: "And when that same awareness, its essential nature shining forth in purity, is as if unbounded, this is known as samadhi." (The "same awareness" is dhyana, described in Sutra III.2: "When awareness flows evenly toward the point of attention, this is known as dhyana.") Samadhi is unbounded by the constraints of time and space. When we experience samadhi, duality disappears. We enter the stream of awareness, where there is no separation between what we perceive and ourselves. In samadhi, our beliefs about ourselves and the world and our habitual patterns temporarily disappear, so that they no longer separate us from the vastness of our true mind.

Samadhi cannot be practiced. Rather, it is available to us in each moment. Samadhi is like a river running concurrently with our ego-based lives. In the same way that we shed heavy clothing in order to jump into a river, we must let go of our deeply held beliefs and judgments in order to step into its current. Like the unfinished sculptures of Michelangelo, we need only to chip away at those parts of our own stone casings—our limiting beliefs—that are not who we are, so that we can emerge in our true form. As the beliefs and judgments that separate us from ourselves dissolve, we become available to the experience of oneness with our universe.

Even though we cannot practice samadhi, we can engage in practices such as the eight limbs. Practicing the limbs builds a foundation that readies us to step into the river of samadhi. When we practice the yamas, we condition our worldly behavior to bring about peace of mind. The niyamas refine our lifestyle to set our bodies and minds on a healthy path. Asana balances the body, so that the mind can abide in a restful environment. Pranayama uses the physiology of breathing to support concentration. Pratyahara teaches us how to detach from our addiction to the external world. Dharana steadies the mind. Dhyana opens us to witnessing presence, allowing us to see reality as it is and to see the illusory nature of our thoughts and biases. These limbs, when practiced and refined over time, lead to the experience of samadhi.

In my experience, samadhi is not something that we suddenly reach and then we get to vacation for the rest of our lives. We visit samadhi from time to time, often quite unexpectedly, and just as quickly as it appears, it also dissolves. I believe that over time, as we continue practicing the eight limbs, the experience of samadhi becomes more frequent and enduring. Still, until we have completely freed ourselves from the identities we've so painstakingly constructed over our lives, samadhi will be an occasional, albeit welcome, occurrence.

But practicing the eight limbs is not about reaching some permanent ecstatic state. Rather, it is about using all the tools at our disposal to be a powerful and positive force in the world. Visiting samadhi is certainly part of this process, but it is only one of the countless steps we will take along our path. Inherent in each small step is the possibility of transformation. Within the painstaking and challenging process of deconstructing our identities lie the jewels of wisdom and compassion.

Sometimes in this process we get to unearth the giant taproot that's been feeding a limiting belief pattern that defines our ego existence. In 1998 I sat my fourth thirty-day meditation retreat at the Last Resort. From the first day, I noticed that my mind was in a state of rampant comparing, not to everyone, but to a particular woman on the retreat that is a cherished dharma friend. In my mind, she could do no wrong—she sat more still than I, she walked more mindfully. I imagined her consultations with Pujari to be filled with wondrous insights, while mine were filled with mundane trivialities. I recognized this comparing as a long-standing psychological pattern that stemmed from being a second child, sandwiched between two outstanding sisters. As a result, I had felt "less than" all my life.

I shared this with Pujari in an interview, and he suggested that I turn my attention to the feeling of being the lesser child. I considered his advice, and then promptly forgot it. One night during the third week of retreat, I was sitting late, after the last bell, alone except for my surrogate sister. The comparing became so pervasive and uncomfortable that I was desperate. I remembered Pujari's advice and revisited my second-child identity. I began directing my mind past the story of inferiority that I'd been weaving for so long to the panoply of emotions simmering underneath the story. Almost immediately, a long-forgotten memory bubbled up.

I was eleven years old. My sisters and I had entered oil paintings of an identical still life into a show at a local fair. My family went to view the show, and I was surprised and thrilled to see that my painting had earned the blue ribbon. When we brought our paintings home, my parents asked me to keep the ribbon hidden rather than showing it off with the prized painting that was now hanging on my bedroom wall. Displaying it would be boastful and might be hurtful to my sisters, they said. I felt undeserving and ashamed of the ribbon. I stuck it in a drawer beneath a pile of papers and didn't see it again for many years.

In that moment of recollection, a lifetime of quashing my potential to avoid causing hurt flashed through my mind. That notion, which I had chosen to identify with, had suppressed literally everything I had tried to accomplish, including my meditation practice. That belief had caused me to sabotage my potential success at every opportunity. Until that moment, I had always thought enlightenment was possible, just not for me. In that moment, I realized: I don't need to do this anymore. Reaching my highest potential will not hurt anyone. It's okay for me to attain freedom.

I felt weightless, suspended in a vastness that had previously been unfathomable. A tremendous burden had been lifted, and my body and mind felt completely unfettered. For the first time, I could acknowledge that my practice was leading to ultimate freedom, if not in this lifetime then in another. Any doubt I had harbored about the paths of yoga and meditation vanished, and it has never returned.

After some time, which could have been fifteen minutes or two hours, I got up to head for bed. Standing at the window, I looked outside. As I gazed at the towering pines, an odd feeling arose: the trees were sleeping. I knew, of course, that trees move into a dormant state in the fall, but now I could feel that they were slumbering. My boundaries had dissolved. I felt completely at one with the slumbering trees, and indeed with the universe. There was no longer a separate "I" observing things. All that existed were the sleeping trees, the starry sky, the sensation of the floor under my feet, the coolness of the night. As I walked upstairs, I felt my body walking itself. I was not even supervising my walking.

I remained conscious through the night, although I believe my body entered a state that might have been sleep. When I arose in the morning, I was still consumed by the vastness. While I moved in and out of the vastness for the rest of the retreat, the boundaries between it and my usual way of being felt transparent, illusory.

Throughout the retreat, a mental image would arise from time to time in my meditations, a vision of my being enclosed by a small brick edifice. As time went by, each time the image returned I noted that some of the bricks would be missing. At one point the roof disappeared. Brick by brick, the building's walls continued to dismantle themselves until that night, when what was left of them tumbled down completely.

No matter how lofty our definitions of ourselves, like my imagined brick edifice, they confine us. The thought that we are anything—whether we think we are entitled or unworthy, beautiful or ugly, good or bad—obscures our vision of who we really are, the unbounded, settled mind. All definitions are manifestations of ego and are no more weighty than any other thought. The only power they have is the power we give them.

Finally, after many years of meditation practice, 99 percent of which had consisted of slogging through unhealthy psychological patterns, I had found the root of the pattern that fed all the others and had begun the process of severing it. Letting go of this deeply rooted self-made identity, at least temporarily, opened me to the experience of freedom. Since that time, samadhi experiences have been more frequent. My pattern of suppression still appears often, but now I see it, and sometimes I catch it in time to stop it from playing itself out.

I believe the process of awakening is gradual for most of us. We have occasional flashes of samadhi, whether we practice yoga, meditation, prayer, hiking, writing, raising children, baseball, lovemaking, or anything or nothing at all. As we collect our energies toward awakening, samadhi appears more frequently and for longer times.

Samadhi arises when we allow ourselves to let go of everything—those illusory beliefs about the world around us and about ourselves that obscure our view and make us feel isolated. What beliefs shape your self-identity? Do any of them no longer serve you? What would it take to considering letting them go? You have everything to gain and nothing to lose.

Afterword: No Expectations: You Can't Always Get What You Want

I N THE MONTHS before I turned nine, my older sister Martha became a master of the yo-yo. Not only could she keep her disc yo-yoing for what seemed like forever, she could perform clever tricks like "walking the dog" and "around the world." As she became more accomplished, she got one of Duncan's really fancy yo-yos, an ultramodern disc that looked like a shiny blue flying saucer. I was extremely envious. Even though I couldn't sustain basic yo-yoing for more than a couple of rounds, let alone accomplish fancy tricks using Martha's yo yo, I was convinced that if I had my own disc I'd be able to rise to her level in a few years.

I made it clear to my parents that all I wanted for my birthday was a yo-yo. I was confident that my repeated requests would get the point across, especially since I'd only asked for one thing. On the big day, my parents approached me with a question: "Would you like to have a yo-yo, or would you rather have a surprise we've got for you?" I really wanted the yo-yo, but I knew the correct answer to the question. So I opted for the surprise. My parents had bought me a Lorée oboe, an instrument that is the choice of most professional oboe players in the country.

At the time, I didn't quite know what to think, especially since I didn't even know what an oboe sounded like. But in retrospect, I can safely say that had I made the other choice, I would likely not still be performing yo-yo tricks. Playing the oboe continues to be one of the great joys of my life, and it sure helps to have a nice instrument.

Perhaps this incident prepared me for my chosen path. As I reflect on my spiritual journey so far, it's safe to say that the most life-changing insights have occurred in completely unpredictable ways—reaching for a doorknob, feeling pain in my shoulder, applying what I thought was heroic effort until nausea arose. The things I thought I wanted from my practice have paled in comparison to the actual gifts I've received. I've learned not to expect anything in particular from practice, because I now know that my most profound understandings were beyond my capacity to imagine until they happened. I've learned to let go of expectations and allow the process to unfold in its own rhythm.

I've also found that because the process has been mostly gradual (with the exception of a few major jolts), nothing has presented itself that I could not handle, even though I certainly doubted it at times. The insight required to untangle some of the more complicated knots in my psyche has always appeared at just the right time. Continued practice of the eight limbs of yoga has provided the stable foundation I needed to stay with it, even when obstacles seemed insurmountable. I've learned to trust the process and to stay out of its way.

One more story:

The Last Resort held its first thirty-day vipassana retreat in 1992. Besides being somewhat overwhelmed by the prospect of a month on the cushion, I came to the retreat in a state of agitation I could not place. On the first day, Pujari gave the instruction that we practice metta (loving kindness) each day at a time of our choosing. I was fairly familiar with metta practice, having sat a ten-day metta retreat with Steven Smith and Michele McDonald-Smith a year before. Still, every time I tried to begin my metta practice by sending good will to myself, it came up flat and dry. The best way to jump-start the feeling was to skip myself and focus on someone else, usually my cat. My frustration with metta practice, with all its attendant judgments, continued for several weeks.

One night we listened to a discourse by a meditation teacher from Insight Meditation Society. The talk's subject was self-love and why it is so difficult for us to generate it. Throughout the tape, a mix of emotions that defied definition spilled out of me. I felt relief, sadness, grief, recognition, and remorse, among many others. A dam had broken, and there was no stopping the river of emotion that coursed through me.

After the discourse, I went to the bathroom to brush my teeth. When I looked at my face in the mirror, I saw the face of a one-year-old child. Instantly I could see the goodness and love that was at the core of my being. I was flooded with a love more intense than anything I had ever felt. At the same time, I felt remorse for how shabbily I had treated myself throughout my life. In that moment, I also understood that the blindingly luminous love I felt was really the core of everyone, and I realized I could never again treat anyone, including myself, with unkindness or disrespect.

For five days I lived in bliss, buoyed by boundless love. Then one night, a few days before the retreat's end, the sledgehammer of reality struck. If I were to live in the light of this insight, my life would have to change—drastically. I wrapped myself into a blanket cocoon and sat out on the Last Resort's deck for a long time. I was engulfed in fear of what was to come. For the first time ever, I contemplated ending my life by jumping off the deck, to avoid the difficulty I knew lay ahead.

Suddenly another thought arose. The insight I had had as a thirteen-year-old about karma and the continuity of life came back to me. I realized that jumping off the deck would not keep me from having to pacify the monster that confronted me. If I jumped, not only would I still have to traverse this mountain in my next life, I would likely have to deal with an additional burden—the karma of having harmed my body in such a violent way. I knew then that I could never end my own life. This realization saved me in the months that followed.

When I returned home, the life I had set up for myself out of a deeply rooted belief in my unworthiness was excruciatingly painful. I could see clearly that my relationship, my job, and even my car fed my life-long assumption that I deserved less than others.

At the time, I was the managing editor of an alternative newspaper. Anticipating a need for some downtime after the retreat, I had requested beforehand that my coworkers not depend on me to pull together the issue whose deadline fell shortly after my return. I was happy to help but did not want to commit to my usual all-nighter to put the issue to bed. Ignoring my request, the publisher, who usually worked with me to meet the deadline, left the production entirely to me while he visited a local bar. I went straight from the airport to work and did not go home for twenty-four hours. I was horrified that this was a life I had chosen.

The publisher happened to be my significant other at the time. The relationship was extremely addictive on my part, the ultimate expression of my second-child syndrome. Before the retreat, I was happy to play second fiddle to his primary relationship, which he had assured me was an open arrangement. After the retreat, accepting only the leftovers of this man's time and energy was unbearable.

I spent the next months in anguish, feeling completely without anchor. All the things I had depended on for security were a painful illusion. Then my boyfriend laid me off because he could no longer pay the bills at the paper. Two days later, I totaled my car. Two weeks after that, I had another accident in the new car I had bought with my insurance money. The oboe I had received for my ninth birthday was stolen. I felt powerless in the face of my addiction to the relationship that was growing less tolerable by the day. Everything I had counted on to give me a sense of identity and purpose was disappearing. For five months, I went to bed every night wishing I would not wake up.

This was a true dark night of the soul, a time of relentless anguish and insecurity. I could not let go of this life I had chosen, but I could not hang on to it either. On the day I finally reached the bottom, I called Pujari. "I have nothing left to hang on to," I told him. "My job, my relationship—everything has collapsed. What reason is there to stick around? I have nothing to live for."

"You're right," he said. "You have nothing to live for if you are depending on your job or your relationship as your reason to be. All these things will someday leave. You stay around in order to live your life fully and completely, to follow your path with loving care and mindful awareness, to learn the freedom of letting go. To develop wisdom and compassion in the process." This was exactly the jolt I needed. In the end, it was the light of truth that cut through my darkness.

A week later, I attended a workshop with Donna Farhi, in which she taught a class on how to generate asana from the internal organs. The class opened me up to a new world in my asana practice. For the first time in many months, I felt a sense of excitement and hope. In Donna's workshop, I knew I had turned a tiny corner. It took another year for me to feel fully recovered.

This period of darkness is not something I would ever have consciously asked for. Like everyone else, I want to be happy. My responses to the anguish and pain I was traversing are not something I reflect on with pride. Like so many significant experiences along the path, I could not have fathomed this level of suffering beforehand. But as I look back now, far from that time, I see that this nadir was pivotal to my evolution. It provided me with a nonnegotiable path out of a destructive pattern. It also yielded a priceless benefit I could not have predicted. Observing my own suffering, and my desperate and unskillful reactions to it, opened me to one of the greatest gifts of my life—compassion for the suffering of all beings.

In retrospect, I can see that the unfolding of this period of my life was perfect. The insight about self-love, followed by the insight about the karmic implications of taking my own life, provided me with the tools to extract myself from a life pattern that could only lead to more suffering. While I would rather have learned these lessons in a less painful way, this is how I had to do it. Not everyone needs to pass through a year of anguish in order to learn their life's lessons, but this was my path. I am eternally grateful for the opportunity to tread such treacherous territory under the guidance of my teachers and with the support of my friends, my family, and my practice.

So, as the song goes, You can't always get what you want, but if you try sometimes you find you get what you need. Let go of your expectations about yoga practice and its rewards. The rewards are far greater than anything the mind can desire. Approach your practice with curiosity and, most of all, with mindfulness. There's no better way to enjoy your life's unfolding than to be present for it. When the lessons come, it's great to be around to receive them. The eight limbs of yoga do lead in the direction of freedom. Trust your practice. The energy you invest will come back to you manyfold.

Resources

Recommended Translations of the Yoga Sutras

Bernard Bouanchaud, *The Essence of Yoga* (New York: Sterling, 1999)

T. K. V. Desikachar, *Patanjali's Yogasutras* (Madras: East-West Books Pvt, Ltd., 2000)

Georg Feuerstein, *The Yoga-Sutra of Patanjali* (Rochester, VT: Inner Traditions, 1989)

Barbara Stoler Miller, *Yoga: The Discipline of Freedom* (New York: Bantam, 1998)

MSI, *Enlightenment! The Yoga Sutras of Patanjali* (Waynesville, NC: SFA Publications, 1995)

Alistair Shearer, *The Yoga Sutras of Patanjali* (New York: Harmony/Bell Tower, 2002)

Swami Venkatesananda, *Enlightened Living* (Cape Town, South Africa: The Chiltern Yoga Trust, 1975)

Recommended Books on Asana

T. K. V. Desikachar, *The Heart of Yoga* (Rochester, VT: Inner Traditions, 1999)

Donna Farhi, *Yoga Mind, Body and Spirit* (New York: Owl Books, 2000)

B. K. S. Iyengar, *Light on Yoga*, (New York: Schocken, 1995)

Judith Hanson Lasater, *30 Essential Yoga Poses* (Berkeley, CA: Rodmell Press, 2005)

Mira Mehta, *How to Use Yoga* (London: Southwater, 2006)

Silva Mehta, Mira Mehta, and Shyam Mehta, *Yoga: The Iyengar Way* (New York: Knopf, 1990)

Donald Moyer, *Yoga: Awakening the Inner Body* (Berkeley, CA: Rodmell Press, 2006)

Vanda Scaravelli, *Awakening the Spine* (San Francisco: HarperSanFrancisco, 1991)

Eric Schiffman, *Yoga: The Spirit and Practice of Moving into Stillness* (New York: Pocket Books, 1996)

From the Publisher

RODMELL PRESS publishes books on yoga, Buddhism, aikido, and Taoism. In the Bhagavadgita it is written, "Yoga is skill in action." It is our hope that our books will help individuals develop a more skillful practice—one that brings peace to their daily lives and to the earth.

We thank those whose support, encouragement, and practical advise sustain us in our efforts. In particular, we are grateful to Reb Anderson, B. K. S. Iyengar, Wendy Palmer, and Yvonne Rand for their inspiration.

To request a catalog or receive e-announcements about new titles, contact us at:

Catalog Request
(510) 841-3123 or (800) 841-3123
(510) 841-3123 (fax)
info@rodmellpress.com
www.rodmellpress.com

Trade Sales/United States, International
Publishers Group West
(800) 788-3123
(510) 528-5511 (sales fax)
info@pgw.com
www.pgw.com

Foreign Language and Book Club Rights
Linda Cogozzo, Publisher
(510) 841-3123
linda@rodmellpress.com
www.rodmellpress.com

About the Author

CHARLOTTE BELL began practicing yoga in 1982 and began teaching in 1986. Guided by her teachers, Pujari and Abhilasha Keays, founders of the Last Resort Retreat Center, she has blended the practice of yoga with that of insight, or mindfulness, meditation since 1986. Following a 1989 trip to Pune, India, she received certification from B. K. S. Iyengar. She teaches workshops and retreats around the intermountain West and has served as faculty at several of Donna Farhi's international teacher trainings in the United States and Canada. Each year Charlotte teaches yoga on women's river rafting trips.

Charlotte has modeled in Hugger Mugger Yoga Products' catalogs since 1984 and represents them at yoga conferences throughout the United States. Photos of her practicing yoga have appeared in *Yoga Journal*, *Yoga International*, and *Shambhala Sun* for more than two decades.

Charlotte writes about yoga, meditation, and music. She has been a regular contributor to *Catalyst* magazine in Salt Lake City since 1998. She served as managing editor for the alternative newspaper *The Event* and edited and produced newsletters for the Intermountain Acoustic Music Association and the Intermountain Iyengar Yoga Association. She has been a columnist for *New York Spirit* magazine since 2001. Charlotte began writing feature articles for the Telluride Bluegrass Festival in 1991 and has been invited to collaborate on a book about the festival's three-decade history.

A lifelong musician, Charlotte plays oboe and English horn with the Salt Lake Symphony and serves on their board of directors. She also performs with the woodwind quintet Scherzando Winds, the chamber folk quartet blue haiku, and the folk ensemble Red Rock Rondo. She lives in Salt Lake City with her partner, Phillip Bimstein, and her three cats. For information about her yoga classes and workshops, visit www.charlottebellyoga.com.

Index

Abhidhamma, 14
activism, ahimsa in, 64
ahimsa (nonharming), 59–66, 70
alcohol, 95
Amaro, Ajahn, 137
aparigraha (nonattachment), 85–89, 101
Armstrong, Stephen, 25, 29
asana, 117–125
  ahimsa in, 64
  alignment in, 122
  aparigraha in, 88–89
  asteya in, 77
  author's first experience, 90
  benefits of, 117–118, 119
  brahmacharya in, 83–84
  breathing in, 45, 46, 129–130
  comparing poses, 124–125
  defined, 14
  dharana in, 151
  dhyana in, 158
  duration of poses, 120–121
  in eight-limbed path, 51
  emotions arising in, 121
  inner stillness from, 36
  ishvarapranidhana in, 116
  mastery of, 123
  mind settled by, 118–119
  mindfulness practice, 28, 121
  pain in, 123–124
  play of opposites and, 117–118, 120
  pranayama in, 132–133
  pratyahara in, 138, 143, 144
  right effort in, 44–45, 46
  santosha in, 102
  satya in, 73

  saucha in, 97–98
  scheduling, 107, 108
  as small part of yoga, 14
  standing poses, 104–105
  steadiness and comfort in, 122–123
  studying books on, 125
  svadhyaya in, 111–112
  tapas in, 107–108
  Yoga Sutras on, 14, 38, 117, 120, 123, 124
asteya (nonstealing), 74–78, 101
attention, 22, 25–26.
  See also mindfulness
authenticity, 25, 27–28, 72.
  See also satya (truthfulness)
awareness, 17, 25–27

balance
  between action and rest, 42
  in brahmacharya practice, 83
  breath and, 45, 132
  maintaining, 44, 45, 46, 106–107
  of nervous system, 118–119
body, mindfulness of, 140–141, 151, 159
boredom, 22
Bouanchaud, Bernard, 153
brahmacharya (conservation of energy), 79–84
breath
  abdominal, 128–130
  in asana, 45, 46, 129–130
  as balance metaphor, 132
  as gauge of balance, 45
  knowing your pattern, 133
  linked to mind, 130–131